Tai Chi for You

Simple Tai Chi and Chi Gung Exercises
for
Daily Health Maintenance

**A Tai Chi and Chi Gung-based programme as part
of a pro-active approach to health and well-being**

P J Farrell

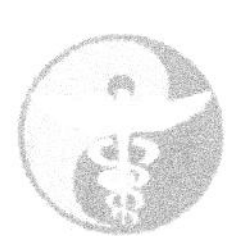

First Published 2018
2nd edition 2021

LIABILITY INFORMATION

The information presented in this book is not intended as medical advice and should not be perceived as a substitute for necessary and appropriate treatments by a qualified medical practitioner. The decision to utilise the methods presented is solely the choice and responsibility of the reader and if embarked upon should be performed gently and with appropriate care. The author, publisher, agents, and distributors accept no liability for any loss, damage or injury caused directly or indirectly from use of this book.

Dedicated to all my kind family

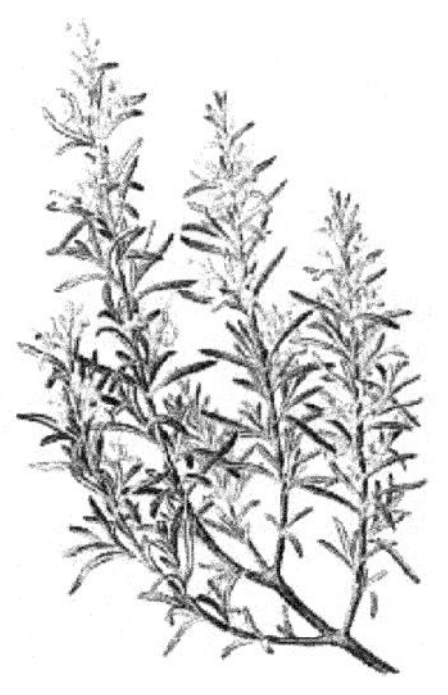

CONTENTS

HEALTH AND SAFETY

The following exercises and information are provided to assist optimum health maintenance. It is always preferable to seek out an experienced teacher. If you intend to embark on any programme of fitness or exercise, including Tai Chi/Chi Gung, you should ensure that you perform the exercises within your own physical limitations and capabilities. If you have any pre-existing medical conditions that might be made worse by practise, obtain clarification regarding suitability from a relevant health-care provider. In any event, pay attention to Appendix 4 prior to practise.

ACKNOWLEDGMENTS

I am indebted to my Gung Fu teachers, particularly the late Rose Li, from whom, over forty years ago, I learned the basics of "Peking" Tai Chi (So named at the time by Miss Li - effectively Yang style of Tai Chi).

I am especially grateful to the person I consider to be my Tai Chi Sifu, a polymath of martial arts, Master Bob Melia, for his kindness and patience in freely teaching me the Sun style methods, and ensuring I understood the internal and external aspects of the art. Through Bob I was fortunate to have met with, and been taught by, his own Sun-style teachers, so I pay great respects to the late Dave Martin (disciple of the late Sun Jian Yun) and his wife Su Ying, with thanks for their guidance in Sun-style and for their kindness, warmth, and hospitality. Although I met Bob's teacher, Master Lei Shi Tai, on only a handful of occasions during his visit to the Fylde coast, his remarkable skills and teaching have continued to influence my practice and that of my friends in the Fylde Tai Chi Association.

Eternal gratitude to my kind, protective, guiding brother and Gung Fu master, John, the Dai To-dai (senior student) of Grandmaster Chu Siu Woon, from whom I learned a small portion of the consummate traditional system of Chu Gar Hung Kuen. John and Bob's encyclopaedic knowledge of Gung Fu and their dedication to the art are my constant inspiration.

Thanks to my dear friend and senior student Martin Brady for his invaluable contribution to this publication and for his tireless promotion and maintenance of The Fylde Tai Association.

PREFACE

There are many excellent books on Tai Chi and Chi Gung, and this presentation is not meant to compete or conflict with any of them. It has arisen from what is nearing half a century of practise and although I make no claim to the title Master or Sifu, the teachings I have received and the experience developed over this time, along with my knowledge of anatomy and physiology, have provided me with a little confidence to present some of the key exercises for daily practise that have stood me and my friends in good stead over the years.

Other than re-arrangement and re-presentation arising from personal experience and preference, the basic methods and information provided within this text are not my own but that provided by my teachers and sources such as those referenced within this text. Furthermore, because many of the instructional books on Tai Chi and Chi Gung can be quite specialised and sometimes complex, I have presented these exercises much as I teach and practise them. In this way, they can be easily accessed as stand-alone sets of exercise for general health and well-being or for gradual development of an extended daily exercise programme for most types of people. In short, any set may be practiced as a regular routine to good effect but, if you have time, by including more than one form, the effect can be enhanced.

The methods are presented in a sequential and graded manner avoiding complex, esoteric or overly technical jargon, which can often leave individuals who are looking for a regular exercise routine somewhat confused and daunted. With this in mind, I have kept the chapters and description of the exercises as brief and clear as possible, although I have provided some introductory and technical information where necessary for clarification and/or motivation. To avoid complicating the main text on the exercises, additional information that I felt was of interest regarding Tai Chi and relevant to the overarching reason for this project of encouraging a pro-active and personally responsible approach to health have been provided as an extended set of independent but related appendices.

The book's title reflects its purpose. It arose from a discussion with my son Sean, who asked me about the book. I mentioned I was having difficulty with the title and explained that I was attempting to produce a book of Tai Chi-related exercise that everyday folk, just like me, with all their physical and lifestyle limitations etc., could practise on a regular basis, without too much difficulty, to contribute in some way, to a greater or lesser degree depending on personal circumstances, to their health and well-being and help prevent conditions conducive to disease development. He said, "The title is obvious Dad, *Tai Chi for YOU!*" So here is *Tai Chi for You*, I hope that YOU find it of some value as part of YOUR daily approach to YOUR health and well-being, which is in YOUR hands… most of the time.

1 WHY EXERCISE?

"To take medicine when you are sick is like digging a well only when you are thirsty - is it not already too late?"
Qi Bo 2500 BCE

Qi Bo, the physician of Huang Di – the Yellow Emperor, implicitly identifies the need to take responsibility for one's health and, consequently, take effective pro-action (acting in anticipation of disease development in order to avoid or ameliorate its effects) to prevent the need for unnecessary (not to mention, untimely) medical interventions. Importantly, along with nutrition (see Appendix 8) and a personally relevant form of "spiritually-attuned" practice, non-competitive exercise plays a major role in a pro-active approach to health. In the author's opinion (as one might expect) the most efficacious exercises are to be found in the meditative and non-competitive methods of *Tai Chi* and *Chi Gung* (also written as Chi Kung or Qigong – pronounced *Cheegoong*).

There are several reasons to exercise, e.g., general health, body image, self-efficacy, rehabilitation, etc. In Chi Gung, the learned postures gently strengthen, stretch, and mobilise, muscles, tendons, ligaments, and joints and enhance flow of body fluids. It is also utilised in martial systems to develop power and resistance to injury. However, with regard to Chinese medical theory, these methods help to prevent and remove lesions that might inhibit the movement of fluids and, importantly and not unrelated, vital energy known as *Chi*. The slow, rhythmic, condensing and expanding nature of the physical manoeuvres encourage effective flow of Chi and fluids to and from the organs of the body. In this way, the practise of Tai Chi and Chi Gung can help the body maintain an optimal degree of health for as long as possible within the ever-present causes and conditions of ill-health that result from daily life, with which we all must contend. The importance of movement and, implicitly, exercise, was emphasised by the ancient physician Sun Siu Miao who provided a simple metaphor:

"Moving water does not stagnate; an active hinge never rusts".

Ensuring effective movement of muscles and joints ("hinges") along with an efficiently regulated flow of fluids and Chi ("water") to and from organs is an essential element of disease resistance and recovery. There are many muscles and groups of muscle, joints and various tissues involved in the exercises to be shown; it is useful, but not absolutely necessary, to know them. However, to achieve optimum benefit and to prevent injury, it is important to perform the exercises correctly.

So then, a key aspect of these exercises is to maintain correct posture when performing them and, seemingly paradoxically, to be able to relax (see Appendix 7) into any stretch/contraction as much as possible. Furthermore, whilst a degree of determination and consistency is required, one should not be obsessive about the exercises. The aim is to bring about not only a beneficial physical change but also a more relaxed mental attitude. By practising the exercises correctly with appropriate mental intent, we begin to find that life and all our interactions with the environment and other beings becomes more relaxed, flexible and equanimous. As the ancient Taoist master Lao Tzu informs in the *Tao Te Ching*:

"Men [and women] *are born soft and supple; dead, they are stiff and hard. Plants are born tender and pliant; dead, they are brittle and dry. Thus, whoever is stiff and inflexible is a disciple of death. Whoever is soft and yielding is a disciple of life. The hard and stiff will be broken. The soft and supple will prevail."*

So now we will look at some of the methods to help us become "soft and supple" or that at least fend off the development of "stiff and hard" … for as long as possible ☺.

The basic warming up exercises that follow are relatively easy to perform and should be practised regularly and at appropriate junctures through the day - especially if you are seated or stationary for prolonged periods. The more elaborate forms can be practised once or twice a day at convenient points. If you wish to examine the theories of movement, etc., related to Chi Gung in more academic/scientific detail, see *Understanding Chi Kung* (2017) by J & P Farrell.

Chapter 2 contains useful exercises especially for people who might have some difficulties with mobility. Chapter 3 exercises are suitable for those who are more mobile. Chapter 4 consists of a standing Tai

Chi-Chi Gung form now with the second part containing an adapted seated form for people who might have some difficulties with mobility and need to be seated. The Tai Chi training forms shown in chapter 5 are for those with mobility; however, for those with mobility issues, the standing postures can be adapted effectively by a knowledgeable teacher. The exercises in chapter 6 can be easily adapted for seated purposes.

Safety First:
If you are practising any seated exercises, you must ensure your chair is secure, will not move and is not liable to tip over. Also, see *Important Points for Seated Exercises*, pages 60-61.

If you are practising any standing exercises, you should make sure your footwear is safe and non-slip and that the floor surface is even and non-slip. Also see Appendix 4 *Towards a Healthy Routine*, pages 127-129.

2 STRETCHING AND MOBILISING – SEATED

Developing a Good Habit

All postures should be performed slowly and mindfully (i.e., constant awareness of each movement and how you perform it - see Appendix 6), and as relaxed as possible. Initially, as with most training methods, it is best to develop a good habit by performing a manageable level, range, and number of exercises on a regular basis, which encourages a consistent approach. Trying to do too much too quickly, e.g., irregular, or enthusiastic bursts, can prove injurious, discouraging, and certainly does not help to form a good exercise habit. Initially, it is best to perform just a small manageable number of repetitions and then gradually increase the number, but only when you feel ready.

Seated Exercises

The following seated exercises are broadly designed for persons with mobility issues or those who might be seated for long periods, e.g., office professionals. Care should be taken to ensure the movements are kept within personal capacity and limitations. Importantly, correct posture or at least improvement of posture is one of the essential elements of Tai Chi and Chi Gung.

1. Correct Posture.

When shape [body posture] *is not correct, then Chi* [life force] *will not be smooth. When Chi is not smooth the Yi* [mind] *will not be at peace. When the Yi is not at peace, then the Chi is disordered."* (Chi Gung adage cited by Yang, 1990).

Development of poor posture (shape) is a common, yet often ignored, health issue. Inappropriate posture can have a marked effect on the spine and impair the vital neural relationship and interactions between the central nervous system (brain and spinal cord) and the nerves to and from the whole of the body. As a result, function of the muscles and skeleton and internal organs may be adversely affected. Such postural distortions create imbalanced muscular tension and if allowed to continue can lead to a range of poor-health conditions because of compression of nerves, blood vessels and organs such as the heart, lungs, and intestines. Such conditions can often develop insidiously, eventually becoming unbearable when they manifest in what might appear to be isolated structural or organ pathologies, the original structural cause or trigger being given little or no attention unless identified by a practitioner with the skill to diagnose and treat accordingly. Importantly, from the Chi Gung practitioner's point of view, these restrictions and compressions also impede and disorder the flow of Chi or life-force just as they do with blood, lymph, and neural transmission (Farrell, 2017).

Tai Chi and Chi Gung can help one become aware of poor posture and therefore, with even just a modicum of effort, help improve it. Furthermore, these exercises offer effective methods of disease prevention, and perhaps, with the timely support of health professionals, corrective measures should things start to go wrong.

In all the following exercises, the basic principles apply whether one is standing or sitting. In both cases, one attempts to develop or maintain natural spinal curves (see any credible text e.g., Tortura/Grabowski, 1996. p182; https://mayfieldclinic.com/pe-posture.htm) with a relaxed, yet upright, countenance. Throughout the exercises, this open posture of the spine and torso should be comfortably maintained. The crown of the head or *Bahui* (Figure 1.2) should be gently lifted so that the chin tucks in slightly.

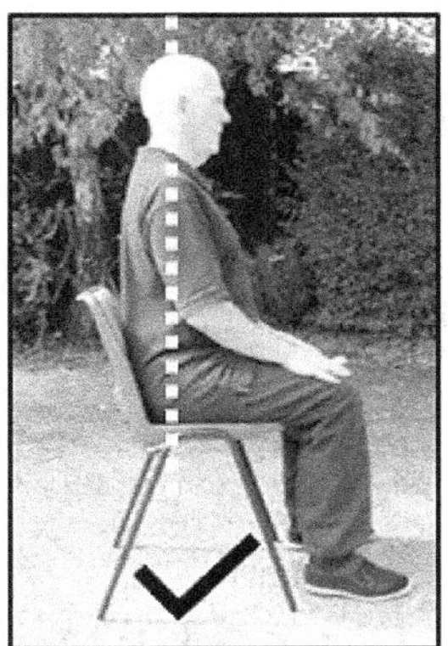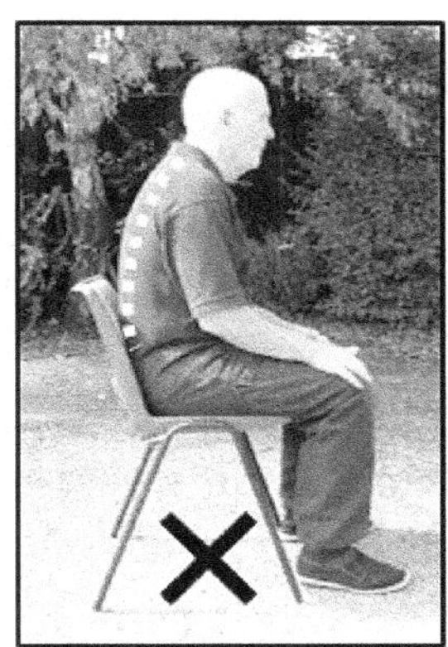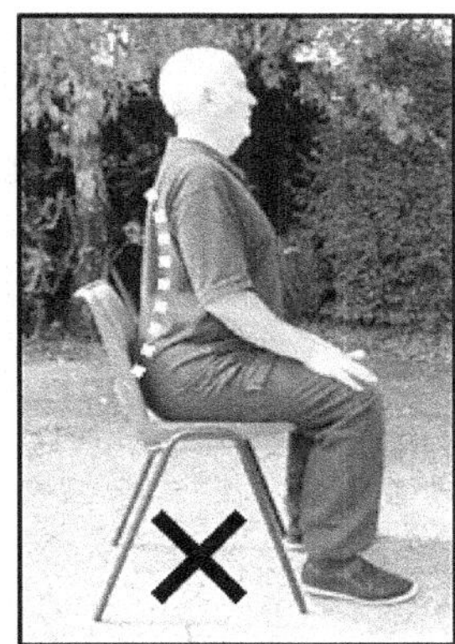

Figure 1. *Correct (✓) and incorrect (x) posture when sitting. The posture should be reasonably straight but relaxed: not rigid. This encourages an opening up and healthy alignment of the vertebral joints and spinal canal. Both feet should be flat on the floor.*

Note that correct posture results not from tucking in the chin *per se* but from the correct positioning of the pelvis and the raising of the *Bahui* which accommodates natural spinal curves. The chest should be relaxed but the shoulders slightly back. This occurs naturally if you feel the shoulders extending laterally with the mental image of an eagle spreading its wing. Figures 1 to 2 describe this positioning.

For clarification, it might be useful here to show correct postural alignment standing. When standing with feet together and hands by the side this is called "no extremes" or *Wu Chi*. Correct postural alignment is shown below. Similar principles apply to seated posture.

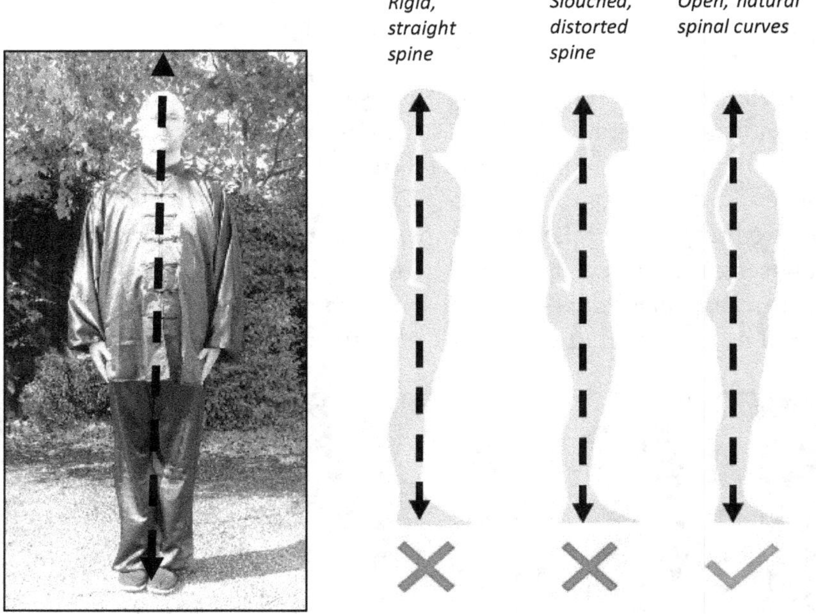

Figure 1.1. *Correct (✓) and incorrect (x) posture when standing. The posture should be reasonably straight but relaxed, not rigid. This encourages an opening up and healthy alignment of the vertebral joints and spinal canal. Both feet should be flat on the floor.*

The crown of the head (*Baihui*) should roughly align with the point between the anus and the genitals (*Huiyin*), which should roughly align with the point between the ankles/heels. Of course, when seated, only the *Baihui* and *Huiyin* align, as in figure 1

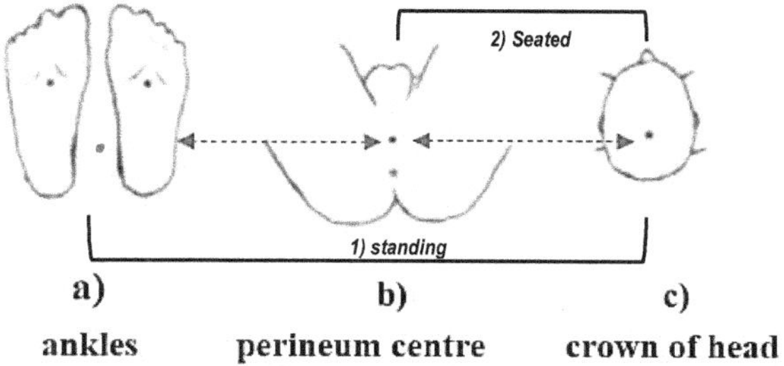

Figure 1.2 *Showing areas that should roughly align when 1) Standing in Wu Chi posture: a) Ankles/heels, b) Huiyin, c) Baihui, 2) Seated: b) Huiyin, c) Baihui.*

2. Relaxing the Breath and Body.

When your posture is correct, gently, and slowly take a slightly deeper than normal in-breath and do not rush to breathe out. This is almost like holding it for a moment so that you feel a slight tension in the chest/torso, then allow the tension to just relax to permit an unforced out-breath. For some individuals, especially those with some form of COPD (e.g., emphysema, etc.) it might be useful to breathe out through slightly pursed lips (like blowing), which can help one relax a little more and fully expel used air. In Chi Gung, we call this slightly deeper than normal breath a "cleansing' breath". This is a little like the deep breath and sigh which we sometimes take naturally following intense thinking or at conclusion of a difficult situation - sort of "Phew! That's that, I can relax now".

Following on from one, two or three cleansing breaths, sit for a short while allowing the breath to settle to a natural inhalation (breathing in) and exhalation (breathing out). To assist relaxation further, when breathing in, try thinking of the word *calm* and when breathing out, think of the word *relax*. These methods encourage relaxed but natural respiration and a relaxed but open body (see Appendix 5 & 7 for more detail). However, following the cleansing and relaxing breaths, we often, inadvertently, lose posture and tend to slouch, so you should readjust your posture accordingly.

There are some breathing techniques that might be incorporated into all the following exercises to better effect, but these should only be practised following direct instruction. In general, following a cleansing breath, one should just try to maintain relaxed breathing* and correct posture throughout the exercises.

There are several types of Yogic / Chi Gung breathing methods, which require instruction by masters in such methods. The method mentioned, although related to them, is used here simply for the purpose of producing consequent relaxion of body and natural breathing. See Appendix 5 for more detail on natural breathing.

3. Neck Exercises.
Note of caution for the following seated neck exercises.

For exercises 3.1, 3.2, 3.3 and 3.4, extra care should be taken. If you have an acute or chronic neck problem, you should avoid this exercise. Also, when stretching and bending the neck, there are certain conditions which can result in dizziness and even loss of consciousness. If this happens to you, then avoid these exercises and in all cases obtain advice from a relevant, qualified health practitioner.

Throughout the exercises, stand or sit with the feet shoulder-width apart in the basic posture and maintain a gentle upward lift of the crown of the head. This helps to open the vertebral disc spaces and reduces undue pressure on the discs and facet joints from the weight of the head during the exercise.

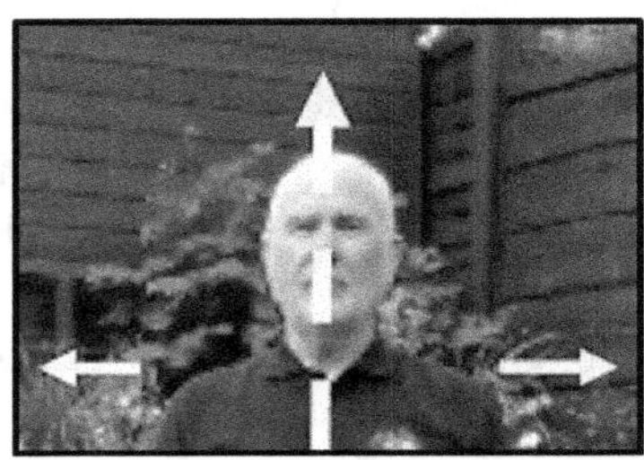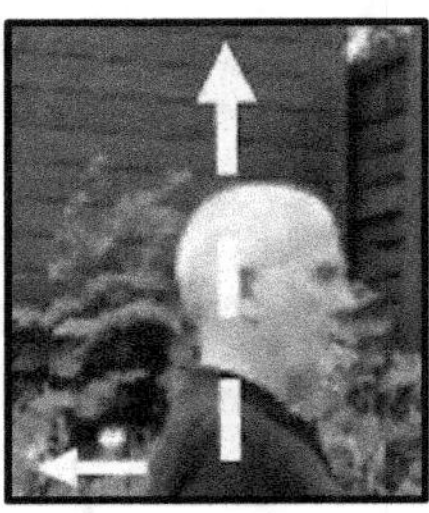

Figure 2. *Shows the ideal head position that is maintained in Chi Kung, which encourages this position in other daily activities. Note that the crown of the head is raised upwards. When this is done correctly it will feel a little like the chin is slightly tucked in. However, once the position is adopted the chin should be raised ever so slightly for optimum 'openness' and to prevent rigidity. Anyone who has experienced the therapeutic extension of the spine by a knowledgeable physiotherapist, osteopath or chiropractor will know the beneficial effects and feeling of release in this extension. The shoulders should be relaxed but level and slightly back, i.e., it should feel almost like they are trying to extend outwards.*

3.1 Turn to Look Behind

Sit with the feet shoulder-width apart in the basic posture. Keeping an upward lift of the crown of the head, gently, slowly, and smoothly, turn the head from left to right. Do not overstretch. Overstretching may result in pain, discomfort, or dizziness and can be counterproductive.

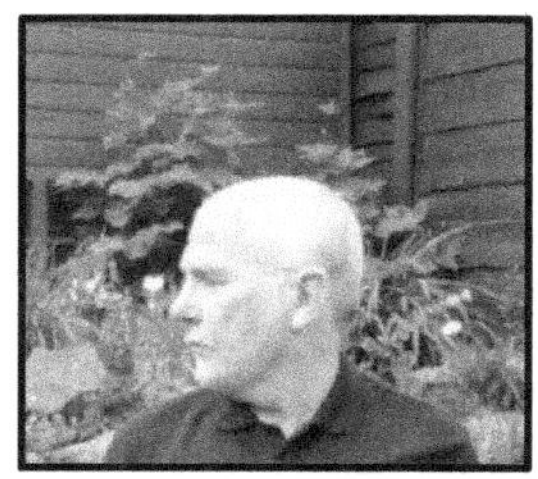 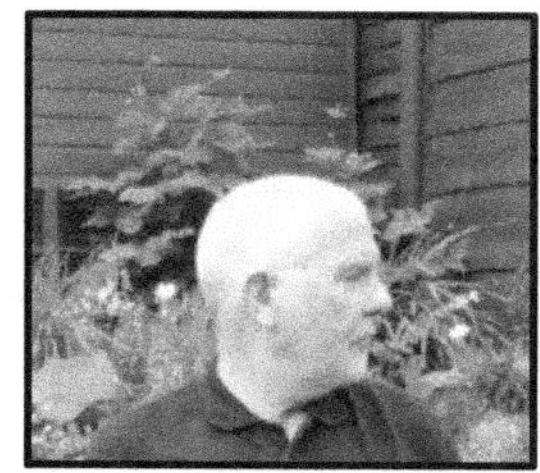

In Chi Gung for health, it is best to keep all movements equal on both sides, i.e., how much you move your head both ways should be determined by the range of movement of the weaker or limited side. Serious neck injury aside, with patience and regular practise, things should improve little by little but in a wholesome, balanced way.

3.2 Look Down into the Sea and Gaze at the Sky

Keeping an upward lift of the crown of the head, lower the chin onto the chest and then look up as high as you comfortably can. The aim is to gently elongate the neck whilst avoiding overstretching, which can result in pain, discomfort, or dizziness. Repeat a few times.

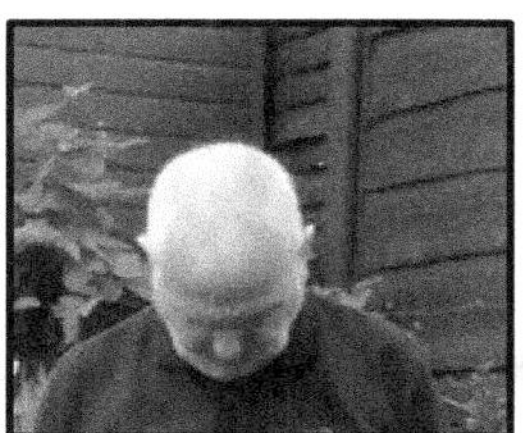 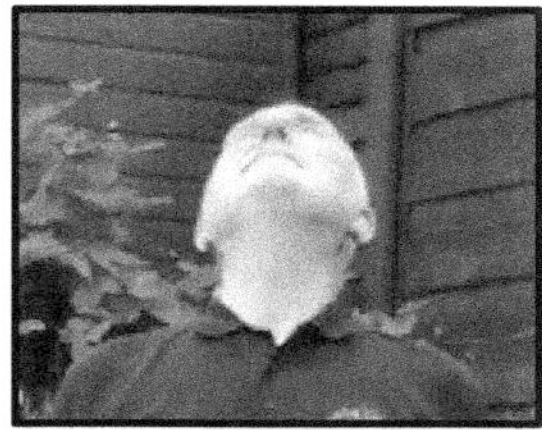

3.3 Raise the Head Upwards from Side to Side

Raise the crown of the head by gently tucking in the chin a little and then push the crown up toward the left and hold for a few seconds. Repeat on the right side. Note that this is not bending the neck to the side *per se*, it is more stretching the neck upwards to the side. Also, there is a tendency to rotate the chin upwards to the opposite side when performing this posture – for the purpose of this movement, the chin should remain directly forward as you gently push up to the side with the crown of your head.

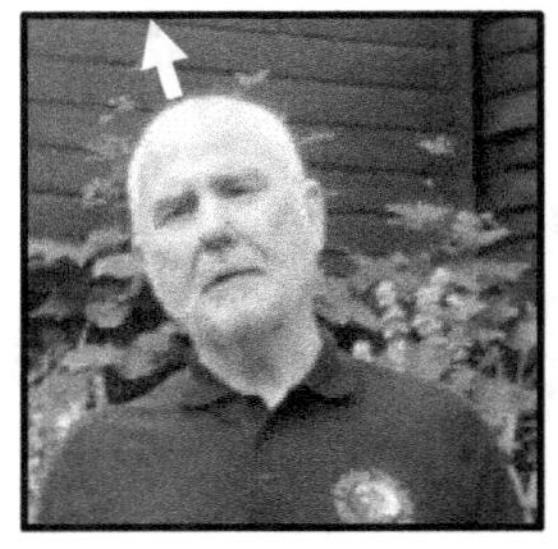 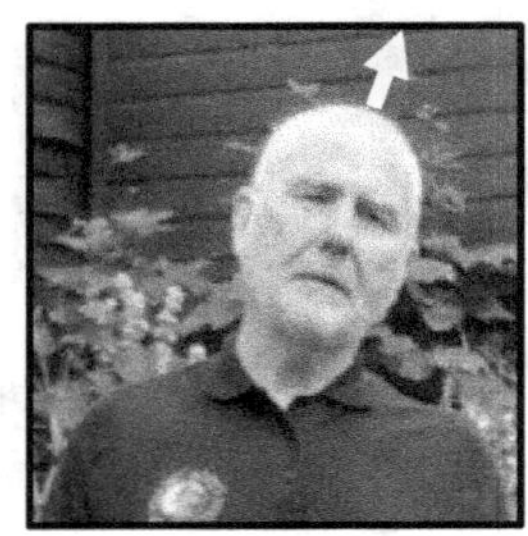

3.4 Gently Rotate the Head

Finally, maintaining an upward lift of the crown, gently rotate the head - first clockwise then anti-clockwise. This movement should feel very smooth and relaxing — it should not cause pain or discomfort. Note that this is not like the sharp and extreme rotation that is often seen when observing athletes warming up. It should be performed in a slow, gentle, and relaxed manner. A useful idea is to think that instead of you actively moving your head around, somebody is holding the hair on the crown of your head (if you have any, unlike the character in the picture below) and gently rocking and rolling your head for you. In this way, the movement will be more comfortable and beneficial.

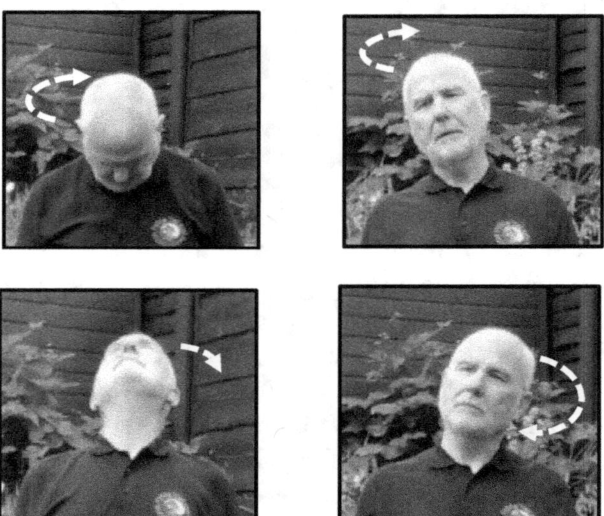

Important — If you experience pain, dizziness or vertigo when performing this exercise, STOP. Get your chosen health provider to check it out it at your earliest convenience?

4. Wrist Exercise.

4.1 With loose fists, keeping the arms as still as possible and the wrists very relaxed, gently articulate both the wrists, or one at a time, as if you were grinding herbs with a pestle and mortar - one way a few or several times, then the other. If you have difficulty circling, just move the fists in and out until the joints become more mobile. You can exercise both wrists at the same time or one at a time.

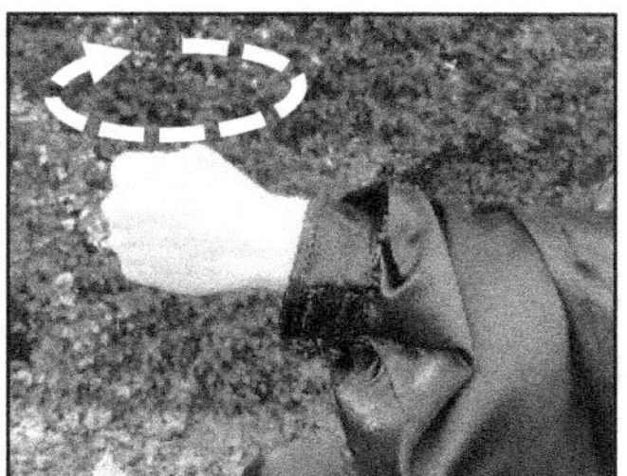 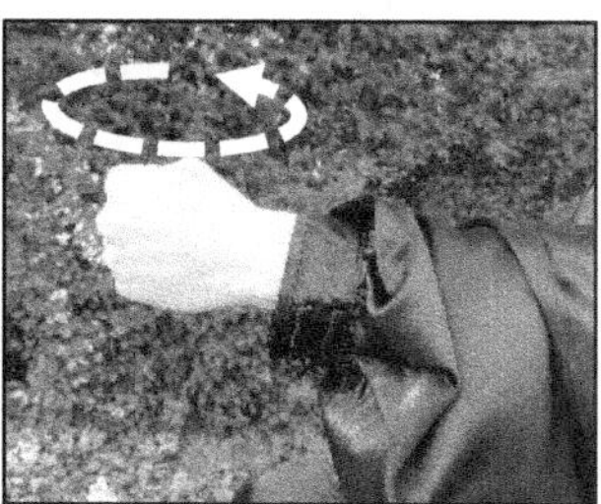

4.2 Now, draw a vertical circle with the knuckle for a greater range of motion. Do this a few or several times, one way, then the other, keeping the wrists as relaxed as possible. You can exercise both wrists at the same time or one at a time.

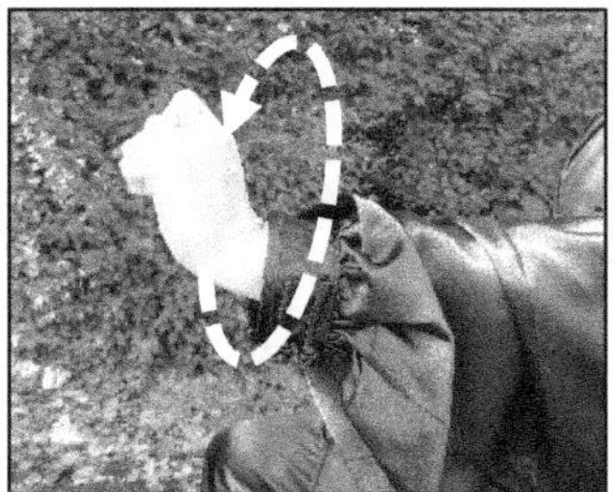 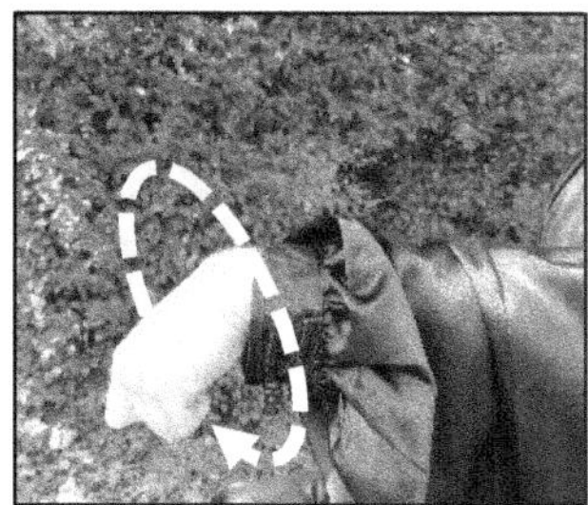

5. Elbow and Shoulder Exercise 1

Slowly and smoothly, horizontally rotate both wrists, elbows, and shoulders like stirring two large cauldrons - one way, then the other. While you do this, engage, and disengage your shoulder blades (bring them together and push them apart, which will also cause an opening and closing of the chest) but keep your shoulders as relaxed as possible.

The photograph below shows only one side, but you should do both at the same time - left, anticlockwise: right, clockwise, then reverse.

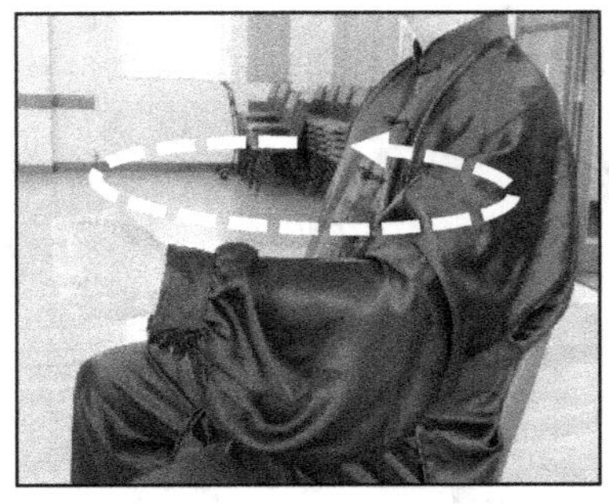 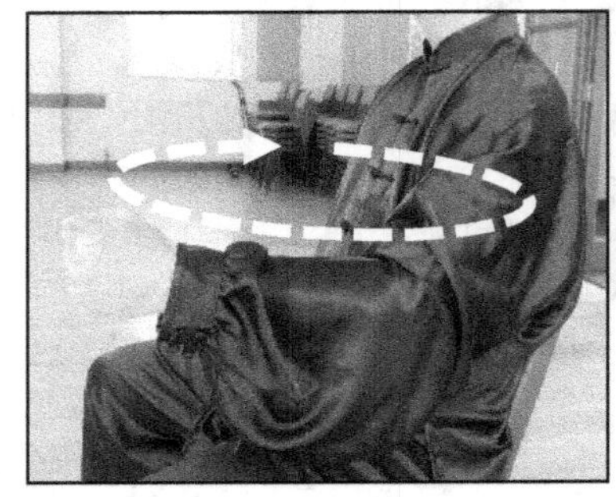

6. Elbow and Shoulder Exercise 2.

Slowly and smoothly, vertically rotate both shoulders, elbows, and wrists like turning a wheel. Turn them one way several time, then the other. Again, you should feel engagement and disengagement of the shoulder blades.

The photographs show only one side, but you should do both at the same time - firstly backward rotation, then forward rotation

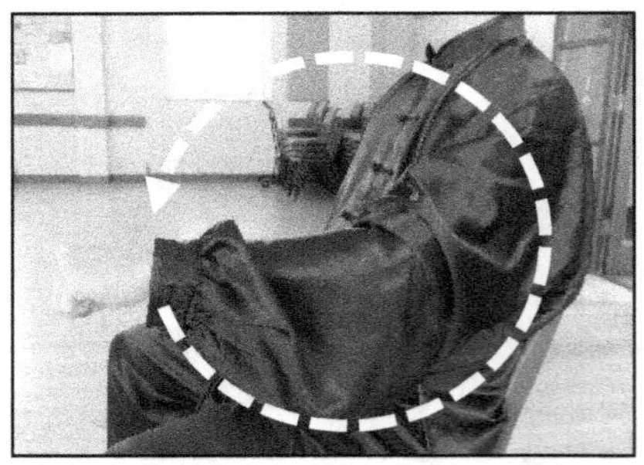 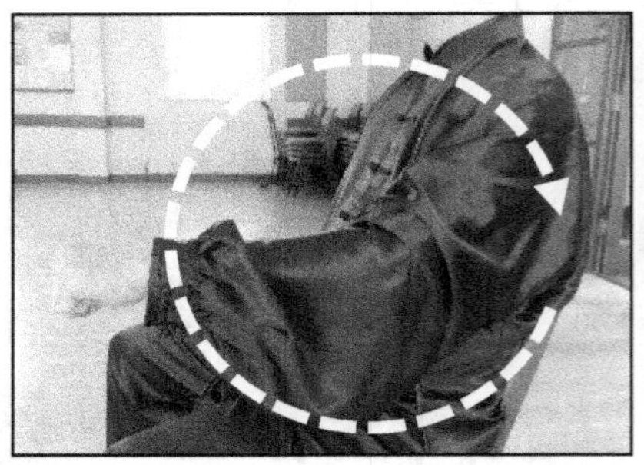

Note that there is a tendency to over-tighten the shoulders when rotating upwards and not to lower them fully. This can case a gross or 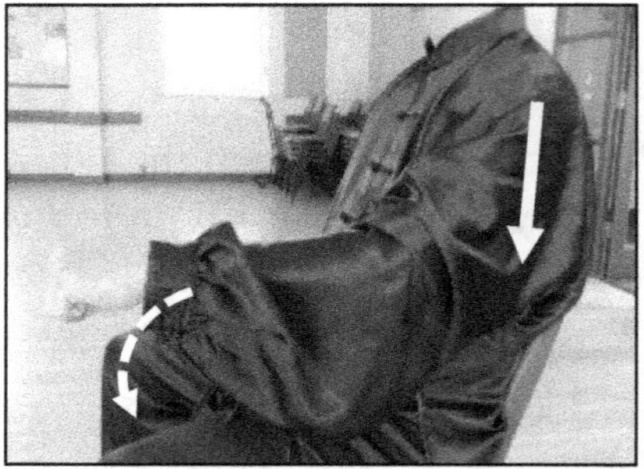 subtle tension to accumulate in the shoulder and neck. One way to help prevent cumulative tension in the shoulders and maintain relaxation is to ensure that you gently but actively pull down the shoulder on the lowering movement as in the photograph opposite.

12

7. Leg / Ankle Stretch.

i) Stretch out the leg and gently pull and push the foot several times to stretch and relax the tissues and begin mobilising the ankle joint. Use method a) if you have difficulty raising your leg or method b) if you can raise your leg. Practise first one side, then the other.

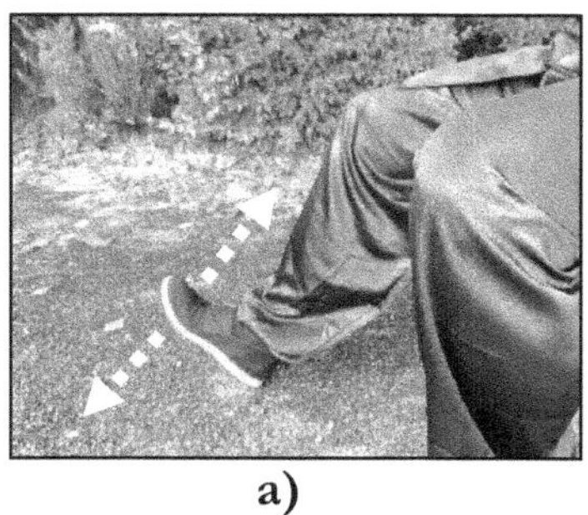

a)

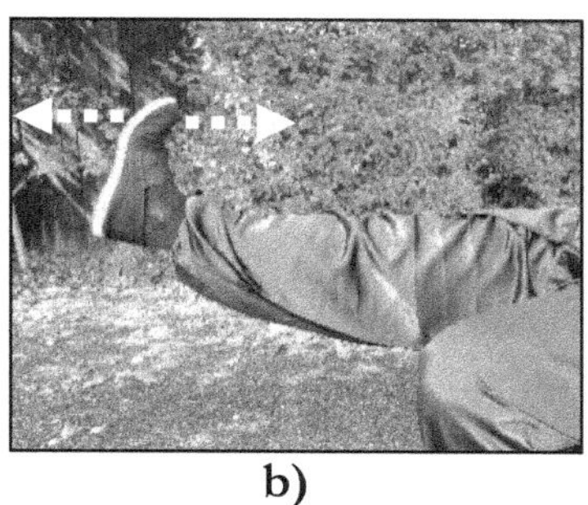

b)

ii) When you have gently stretched the tissues and after you have completed exercise 8.i, you can enhance the movement by pulling back the foot and holding it in the stretch for a few seconds. Within the stretch, try to think about the tension relaxing. Next push the toes forward, again try to relax the stretch. Repeat on both sides a few times.

8. Ankle Rotation.

i) Keeping the leg still, draw a relaxed circle with the toes. Use method a) if you have difficulty raising your leg or method b) if you can raise your leg. Practise first on one side, then the other.

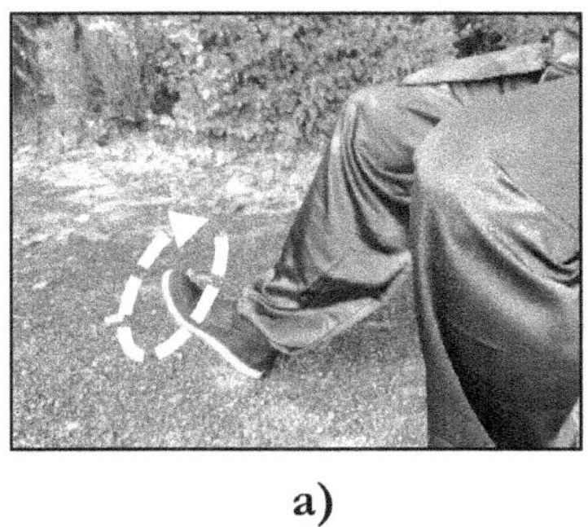

a)

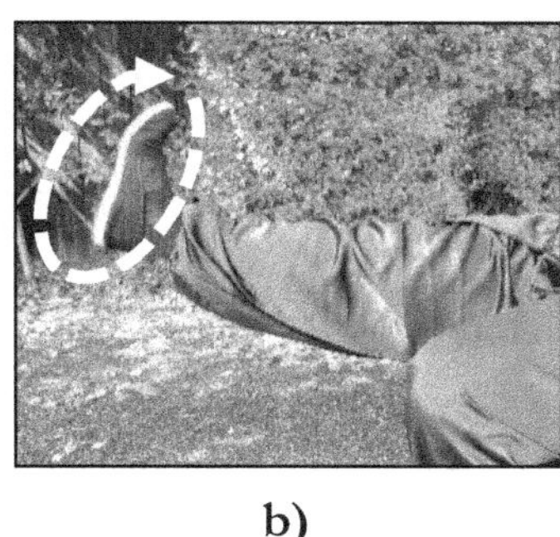

b)

ii) Now that you have gently stretched the tissues and mobilised the ankle joints and after you have completed exercise 7.ii, if you wish, you can enhance the movement by keeping the leg still and then, very slowly and carefully, draw a circle with your toes as large as you comfortably can. Practise circling in both directions.

9. Leg Raise and Stretch.

This exercise can put a little strain on the low back if you are not careful. It is recommended that you support yourself by holding the sides or arms of the chair whist performing the exercise. Raise the knee with the foot tilted upwards then push out the heel. If you have difficulty raising your leg, just stretch it out as far as you comfortably can. Slowly and gently, draw the knee back up then slowly and gently lower the foot with the toes pointing down. Finally, gently rest the foot on the floor. Repeat a few times, first one leg then the other.

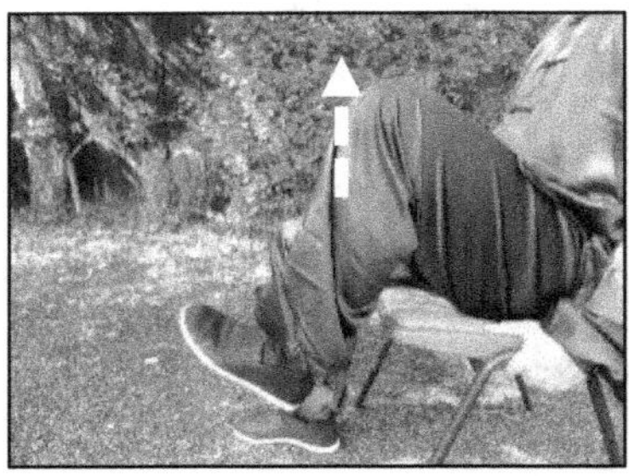
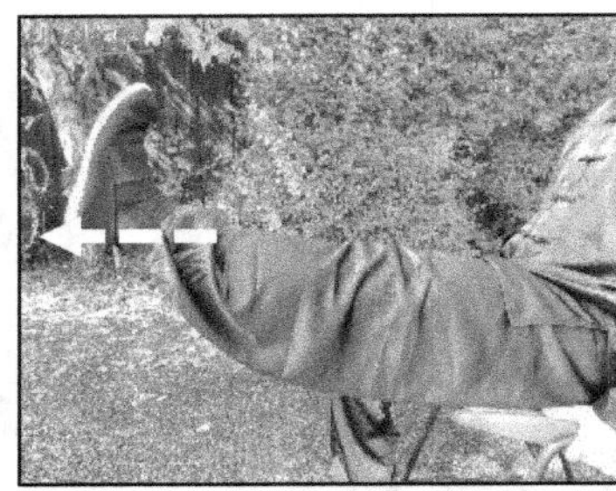
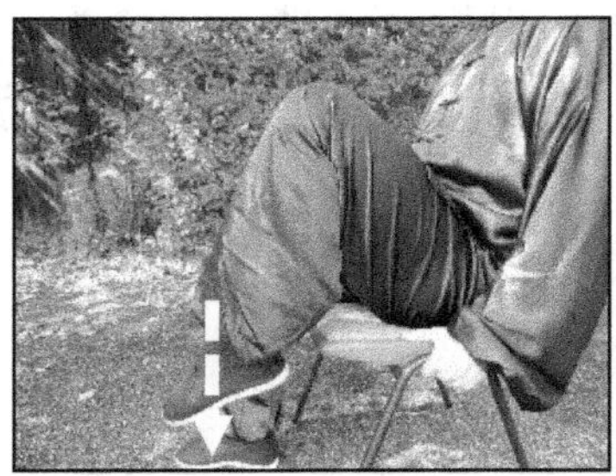

The above exercises are not definitive or exhaustive but contain a broad, yet important, spectrum of movement particularly with regard to Chi Gung and Tai Chi. They are especially important for folk who are sat immobile for long periods. They may be usefully and briefly used prior to standing following long periods of immobility.

3 STRETCHING AND MOBILISING – STANDING

Basic Standing Posture 1 - Upright Posture.

The principles discussed previously apply when standing. Stand with the feet together and hands by your side (*Wu Chi*) then step left to shoulder-width (*Tai Chi*), feet parallel or slightly angled. Draw the shoulders slightly back with the crown of the head lifted so that the chin tucks in slightly. The shoulders should be relaxed with a slight gap under the armpits and the arms hanging heavy and relaxed. The crown of the head should roughly align with the point between the anus and the genitals, which should roughly align with the point between the ankles/heels (Figure 1.2). You should feel a lightness of the upper body but remain strongly rooted – you should be able to really "feel" the ground. Relax the knee joints (slightly unlocked) in line with the feet. This posture is used for starting and when rising up from posture 2. It can be used within the forms should the legs become tired. Structural alignment is important, but the overall feel should be quite relaxed. You should try to maintain the natural spinal curves (Figure 1.1).

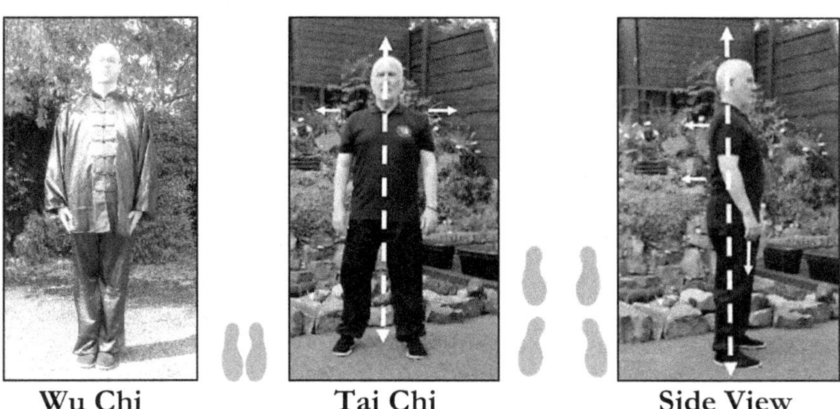

| Wu Chi | Tai Chi | Side View |

Before commencing the exercises, use this position to gently and loosely shake the limbs and body to release general tension.

Basic Standing Posture 2 – Horse-Riding Posture

Stand as in posture 1 but unlock the knees a little more. In this position, you should align the knees with the feet and avoid extending them beyond the toes. If done correctly, you should feel like your pelvis and thighs are sinking into the legs, there should be a gentle sensation of outward rotation of the knees. You should feel the tailbone pulling gently downward, which will curve the pelvis very slightly forward – do not tilt the pelvis forward as this will result in a tightening of the pelvic area. The pelvis needs to be like a basin in which the internal organs sit nicely (a relaxed, yet stable, pelvic area is important for the efficient flow of Chi through certain vessels).

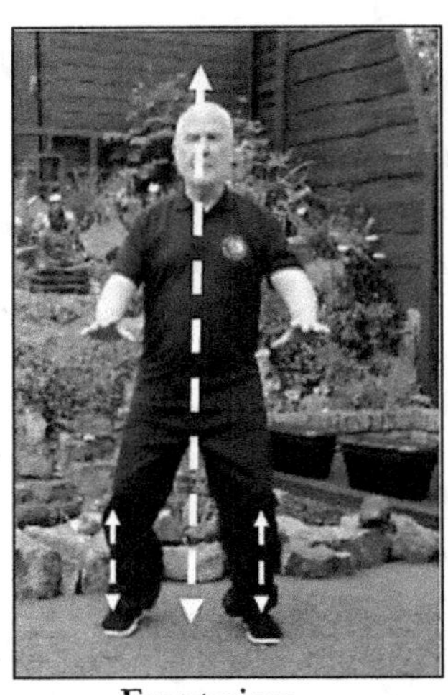
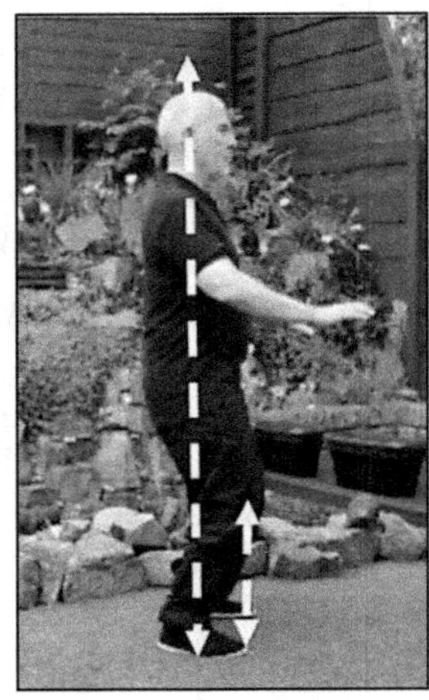

Front view   **Side view**

The crown of the head should roughly align with the point between the anus and the genitals, which should now roughly align with the point between the point on the feet known as the *Bubbling Spring* or *Yongquan* (See front and side view above and figure 3 below). You should feel a lightness of the upper body with a relaxed waist yet remain strongly rooted. Remember, the knees should be in line with the feet and should not go beyond the toes (except in certain exercises).

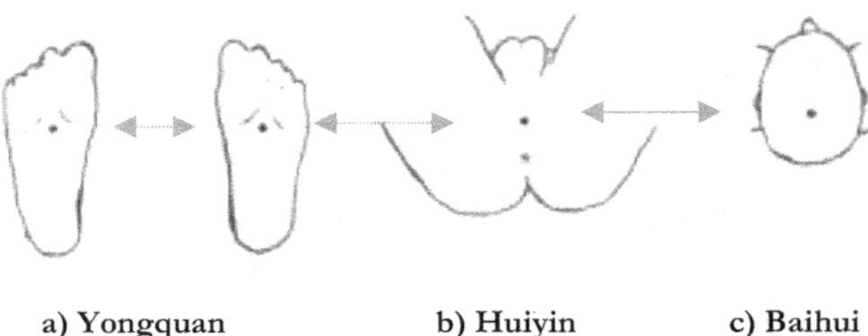

a) Yongquan   **b) Huiyin**   **c) Baihui**

Figure 3. *Showing three areas that should roughly align when in the horse-riding posture:*

Note. The Horse-Riding posture (*Mabu*) might prove a little uncomfortable at first but, done correctly, it will become quite natural and help to develop a strong and comfortable "physical root", which will, eventually, be expressed as a strong foundation within the interconnected, balanced (yin/yang) movement of the exercises.

It should be emphasised here that such posture-training, from the viewpoint of health maintenance, is the essential foundation for the general physical and mental health associated with the practice of Tai Chi and Chi Gung. Correctly adjusted posture and stable physical foundation engenders a stronger and more profound "mental root", i.e., confidence, mindfulness, and clarity. To recapitulate, *"when shape* (body posture) *is not correct, then Chi will not be smooth. When Chi is not smooth the Yi* (mind) *will not be at peace. When the Yi is not at peace, then the Chi is disordered."*.

Basic Standing Posture 3 - Relaxing Before Beginning

Slowly step out and sink into the horse-riding posture. Maintain a relaxed, slow pace and sweep the relaxed yet open palms (Tai Chi palm) outwards and then inwards so that your *laogong* points (roughly the centre of your palms) are facing the lower *dantien* (as in figure 4). You should try to remain in this position for a short while and simply allow your mind and body to rest, not focusing on anything in particular. Just be "present: "standing like a tree" - strong, calm, confident and relaxed.

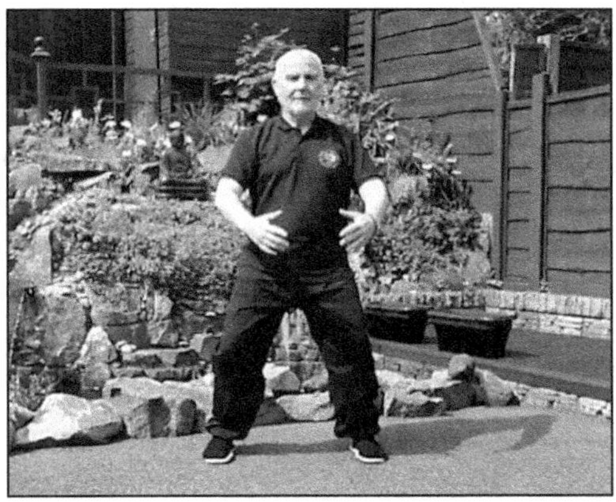

Figure 4. *"Standing like a tree" - useful for relaxing the mind, body, and breath. It is part of the Zhan Zhuang (See appendix 3) set of Chi Kung exercises found in the internal systems such as Yi Chuan and Xing Yi. The palms are quite relaxed and open as shown above.*

1. Arm Swinging

Arm swinging or *Ping Shuai Gong* is a simple, yet efficacious set of exercises. The following arm swinging set has been adapted slightly for warming up purposes, but they provide an easy exercise to practise daily throughout the day to mobilise body fluid, tissues, and joints, and especially assist in fascial tissue (an important connective tissue) health which provides beneficial effects on neural, circulatory, and visceral health and chronic pain.

Stand with the feet shoulder-width apart in the basic posture, and then, in a very flaccid manner, gently shake the body. Now loosely swing the arms forward and back for as long as you feel comfortable. Try to avoid over-emphasising muscular action, keep your shoulders relaxed and let your arms swing in a flaccid and carefree manner. Avoid forceful extension of the range of movement, it will extend naturally over time, especially do not elicit, or exacerbate pain (These principles apply in all the following postures). This set of exercises can be performed slowly or vigorously but always relaxed and carefree. This exercise can be easily adapted for sitting practise also.

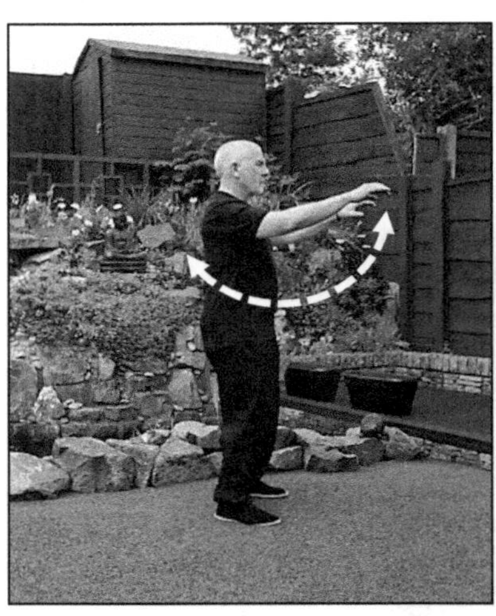 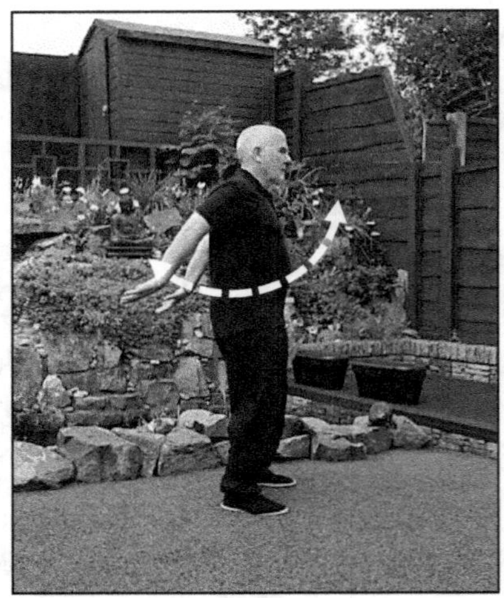

2. Marching on the Spot

Continue swinging the arms but then march on the spot, raising the knee slightly at first and then higher as the muscles warm up and stretch.

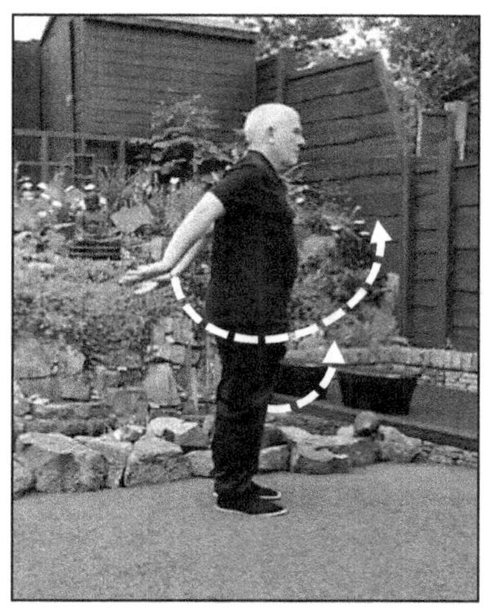 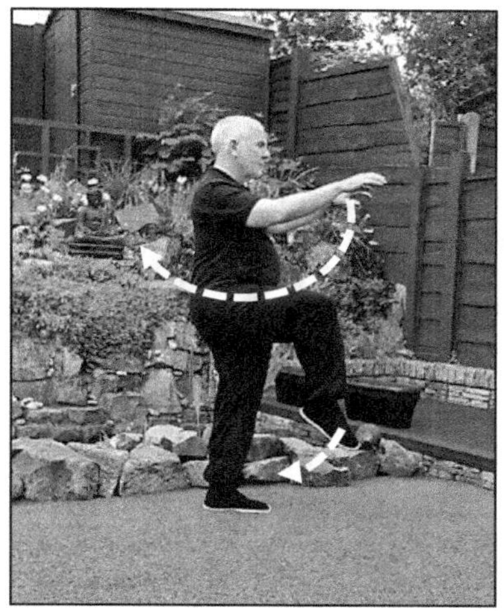

There is a common tendency to draw the knee up in a distorted valgus (knock-kneed) manner with the foot everted (tilted outwards). Practise drawing the knee up straight, in line with the foot pointing straight down (plantar flexion). Let the foot fall to the ground in a relaxed manner but learn to place it down gently without any noise. Alternate stepping left and right in this manner for some time.

3. Reaching to the Sky and Kicking the Tailbone

Continue swinging the arms but throw them above the head and raise the heels up behind, alternately left and right. Keep very relaxed when doing these exercises, the movements should have a playful feel about them.

The kick should be nice and free. Keep the knees close and aim the heel for the backside/tailbone. Try to avoid flexing the hip and drawing the knee up. You should feel the hip extend.

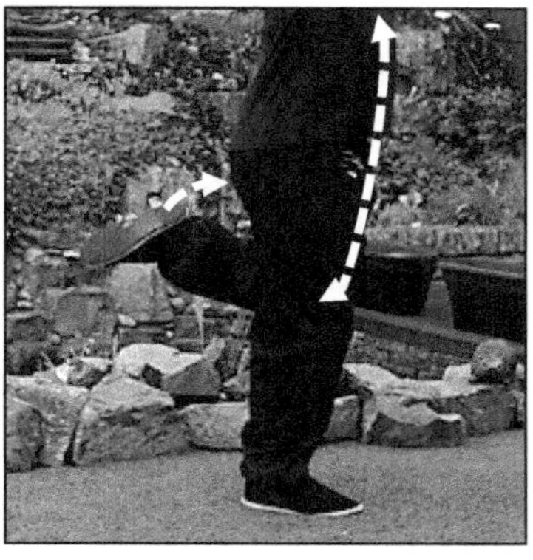

One aim is to feel a healthy stretch of the whole of the front of the thigh and torso with a degree of hip extension.

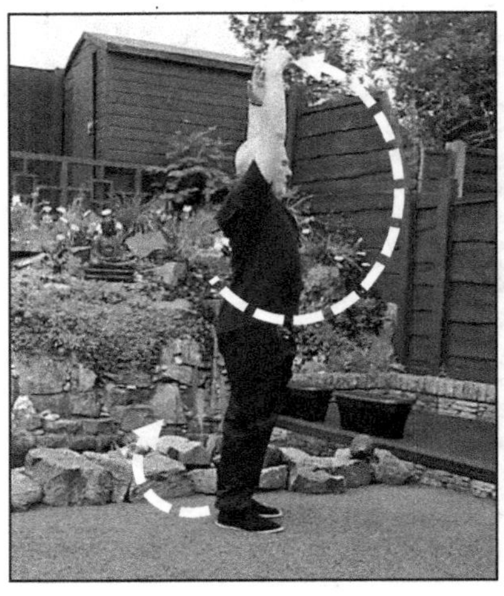 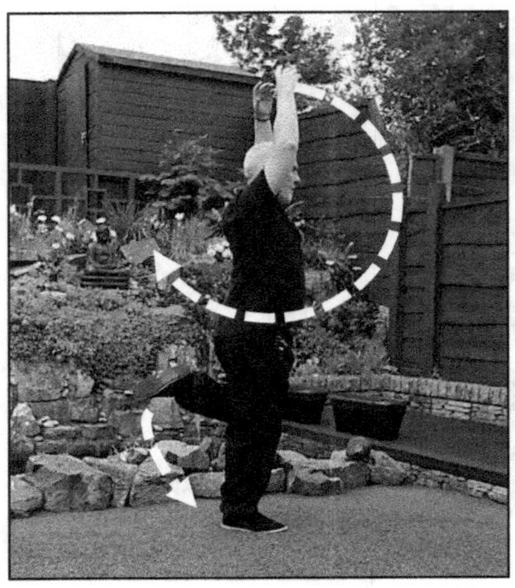

4 - Arm Swinging and Rise on the Toes

Return to swinging the arm by the side but now raise the heels up and down in coordination with the arm-swing.

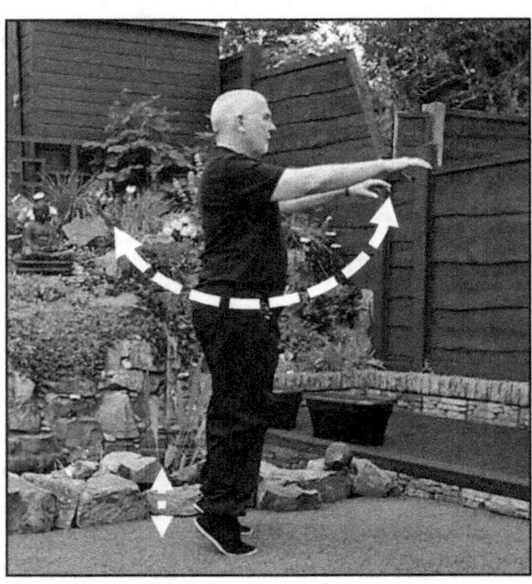

There is a common tendency to throw the heels out when rising. Instead, you should rise on the balls of the feet and toes but try to distribute pressure over all the toes without allowing the heels to tilt outwards.

Although this exercise is useful for most people, if you suffer from foot conditions such as *plantar fasciitis* or *Morton's neuroma,* it might exacerbate the problem, so you should avoid the rising on the toes and instead seek advice from a relevant, qualified health practitioner with regard to specific exercise / treatment.

5 - Playing the Damaru (Tibetan drum)

Stand in the horse-riding posture and gently rotate your body at the waist. You should keep the waist relaxed as you do this. Gradually, allow the arms to swing loosely in a flaccid manner.

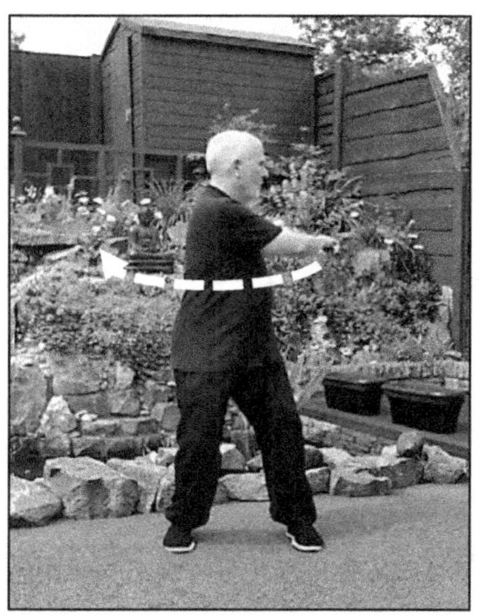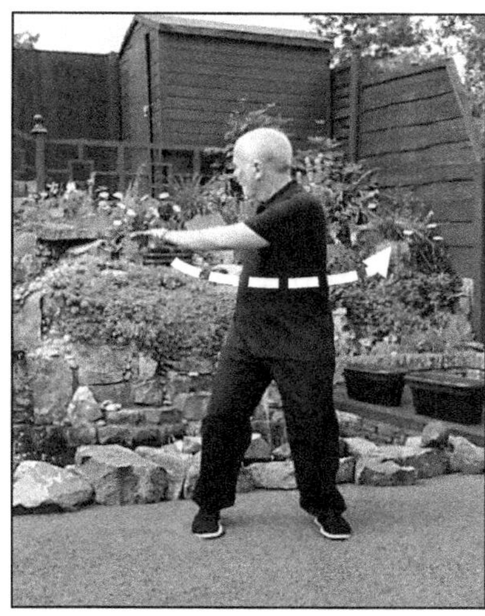

Try to maintain a strong horse-riding posture and avoid the tendency to twist the thighs/knees. Furthermore, there is a tendency to allow the low back (lumbar spine) to extend (bend backwards) to compensate for limited rotation, try to avoid this by keeping the low back pushed out slightly (i.e., maintain proper natural spinal curves).

When your leg and knee strength develop, you can begin to practise weight transfer from one leg to the other as you swing the arms but ensure that your hip knee and foot alignment of the weight bearing leg is correct (commonly, but incorrectly, the weighted hip pops outwards). When you are more experienced, you can incorporate a weight/stance shifting technique from *Xing Yi,* moving the body from left to right, but it is best to have some direct instruction on how to do this. If you have an extended interest in the Chi Gung theory of this and similar types of exercise, see Frantzis (1993).

Note of Caution for the Following Standing Neck Exercises

For exercises 6, 7, 8 and 9, extra care should be taken. If you have an acute or chronic neck injury you should avoid this exercise. There are certain conditions which can result in dizziness and even loss of consciousness when stretching and bending the neck. If this happens to you, then avoid these exercises and obtain advice from a relevant, qualified health practitioner.

Reminder

In all these neck exercises, to avoid undue pressure on areas of the joints, maintain a gentle upward lift of the crown. If done correctly, it should result in a gentle tucking in of the chin (see Figure 2).

6. Turn to Look Behind

Stand with the feet shoulder-width apart in the basic posture. Raise the crown of the head by gently tucking in the chin a little and turn the head gently left and right. For the following neck exercises, apply the principles mentioned earlier in the section on seated exercise.

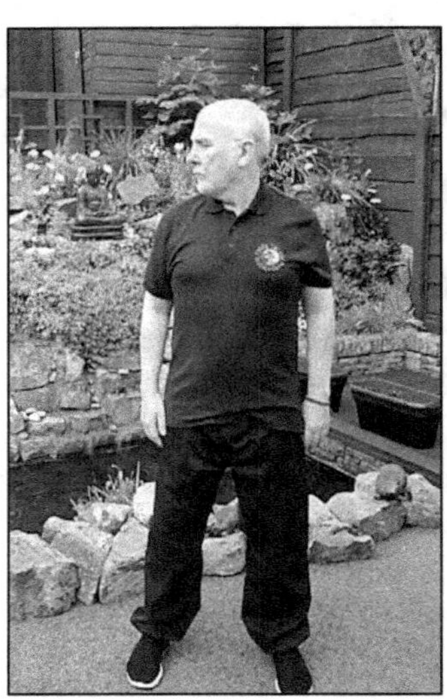 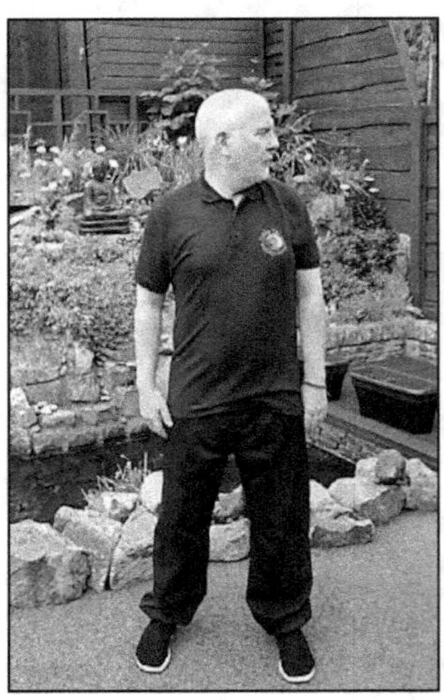

It is important not to force these neck exercises. In Chi Gung it is sufficient to repeat movements while maintaining a gentle and balanced approach. For example, if movement one way is limited then that is as far as you need to go. However, the movement on the good side should only be the same as the limited side. Serious neck issues that require treatment aside, things will improve, gradually.

7. Look Down into the Sea and Gaze at the Sky

Again, using the principles mentioned earlier, lower your chin onto the chest and then tilt the head backwards to look up. Repeat.

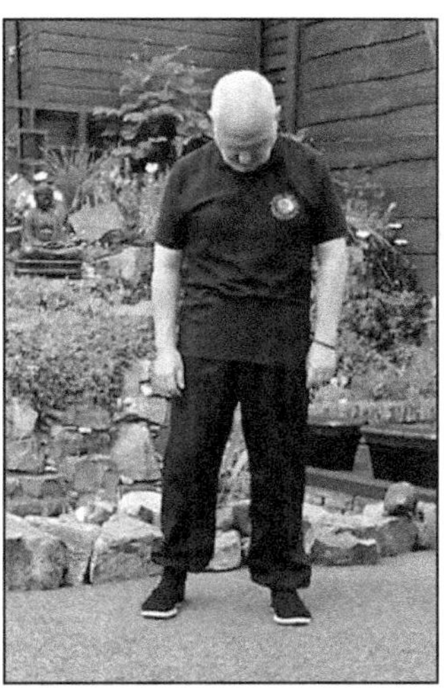 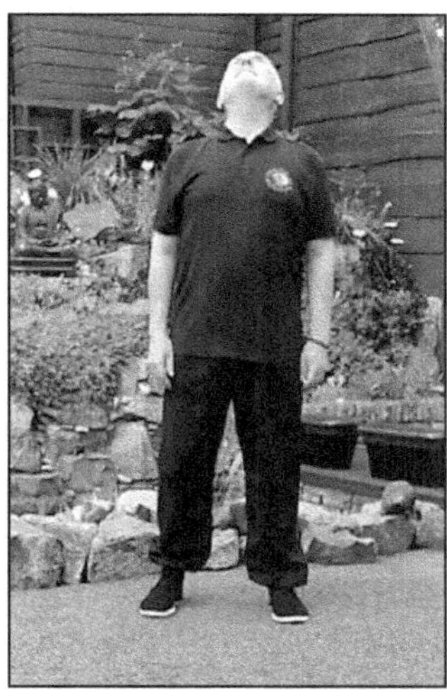

8. Raise the Head Upwards from Side to Side

Stand with your feet shoulder-width apart in the basic posture. Raise the crown of your head by gently tucking in the chin a little and then push it up toward the left and hold for a few seconds then do the same on the right. Repeat a few times

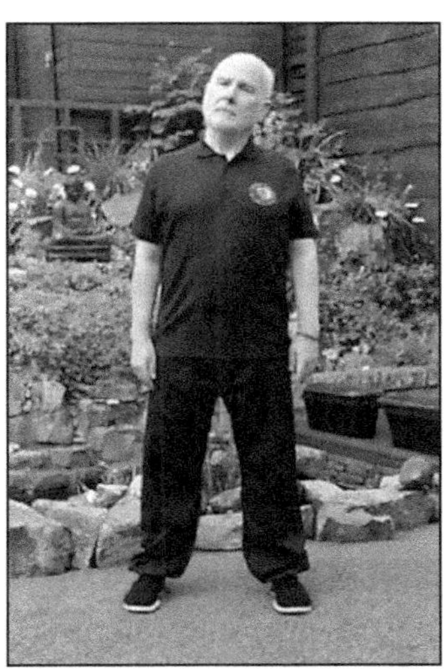 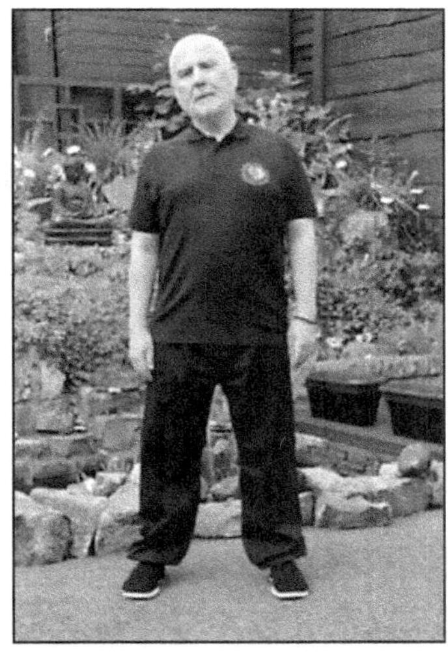

9. Gently Rotate the Head

Using the principles mentioned in Chapter 2, carefully, but in a relaxed manner, rotate your head, clockwise a comfortable number of times, then anti-clockwise (see seated exercise 3.4).

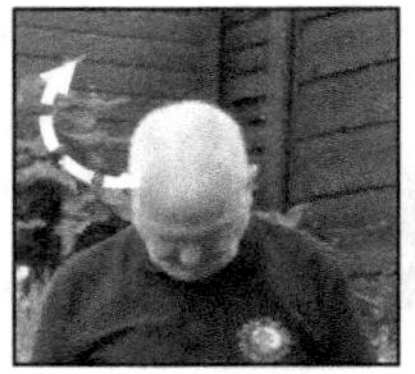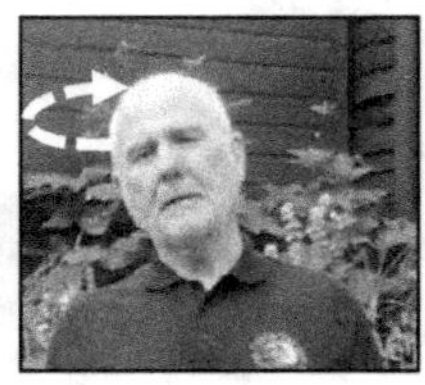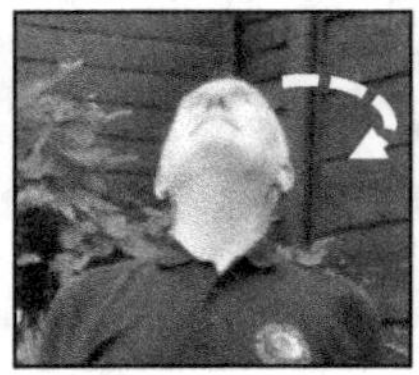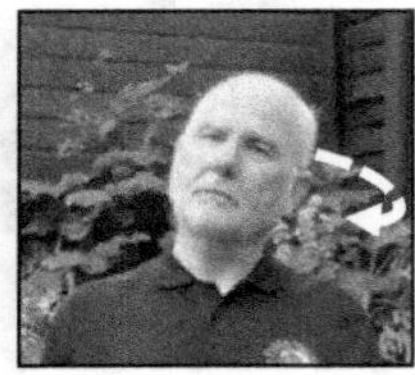

10. Wrist Exercise.

10.1 With loose fists, keeping the arms as still as possible and the wrists very relaxed, gently rotate your wrists like grinding herbs with a pestle and mortar; one way a few or several times, then the other. You can exercise both wrists at the same time or one at a time.

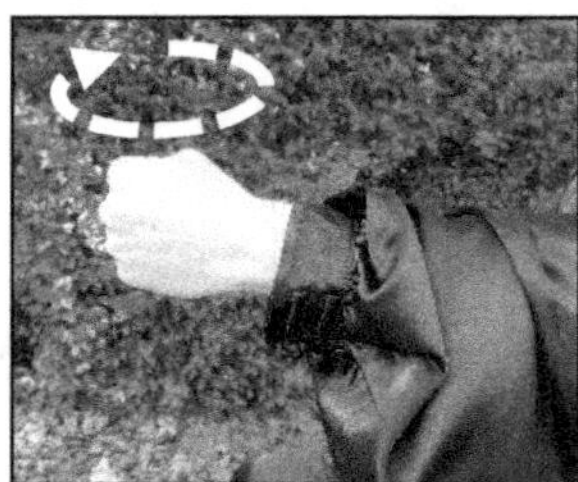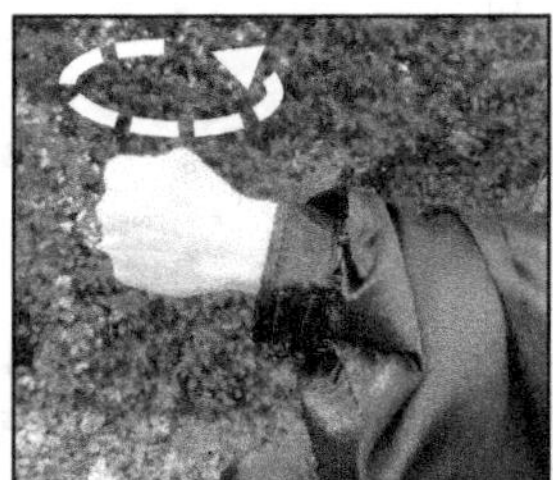

10.2 Now using both wrists, draw a vertical circle with the knuckles for a greater range of motion. Do this a few or several times, one way, then the other, keeping the wrists as relaxed as possible. You can exercise both wrists at the same time or one at a time.

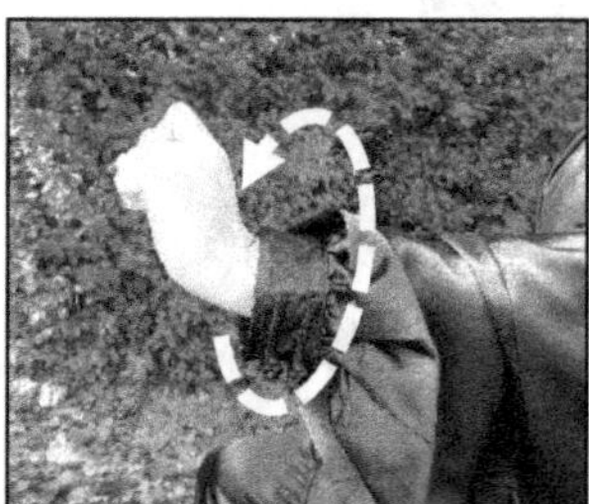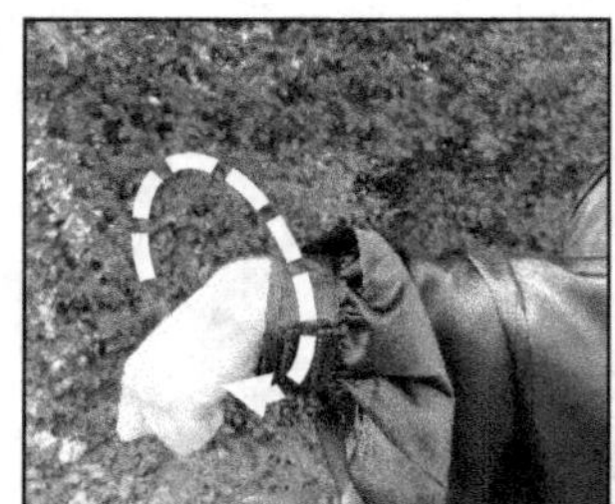

11. Elbow and Shoulder Exercise 1

Using the principles mentioned earlier, horizontally rotate both wrists, elbows, and shoulders like stirring two large cauldrons: several times one way, then several times the other. You should notice an engagement and disengagement of the shoulder blades as you do this.

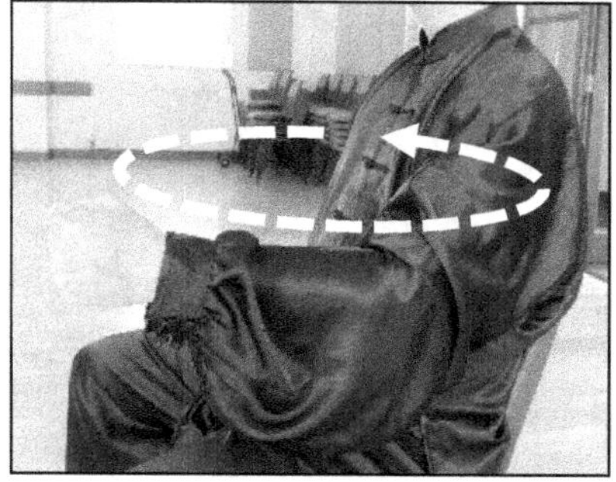

The photograph shows only one side, but you should do both sides at the same time - left, anticlockwise: right, clockwise, then vice-versa

12. Elbow and Shoulder Exercise 2.

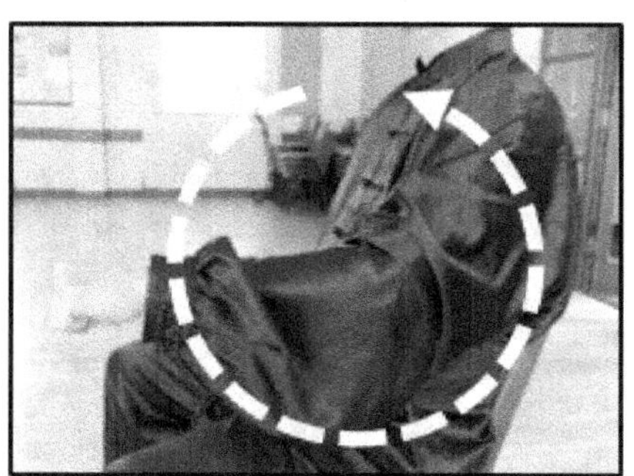

Vertically rotate both shoulders, elbows, and wrists like turning a wheel; one way then the other. Keep the shoulders as relaxed as possible when you are raising them and try to lower them all the way down. Again, you should feel engagement and disengagement of the shoulder blades

The photograph above shows only one side, but you should do both sides at the same time - firstly backward rotation, then forward rotation as shown in seated exercise 6.2.

13. Rotate the Mill Wheel

Stand with the feet shoulder-width apart in the basic posture. Raise your hands and <u>stretch upward</u> then rotate to the left and <u>relax downward</u>, then stretch back up. Rotate first clockwise, then anti-clockwise. Unless you have strong back-muscles and are very flexible, you should bend your knees when relaxing downwards.

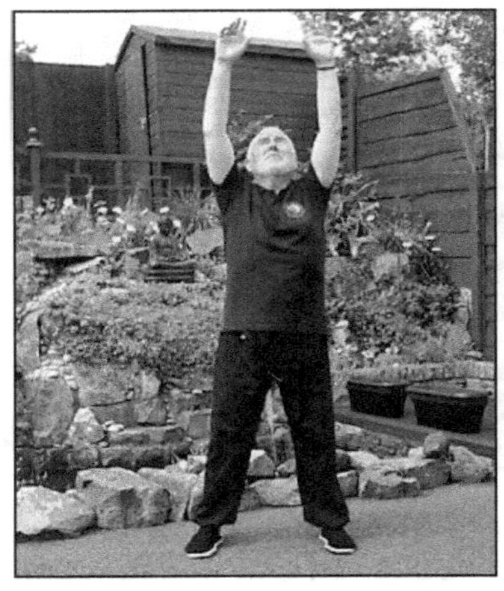
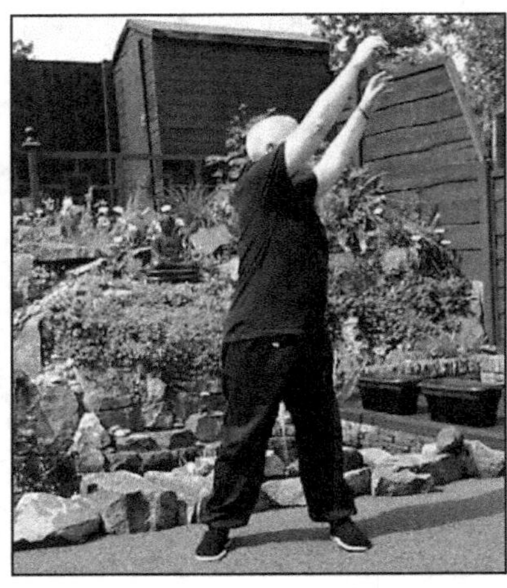

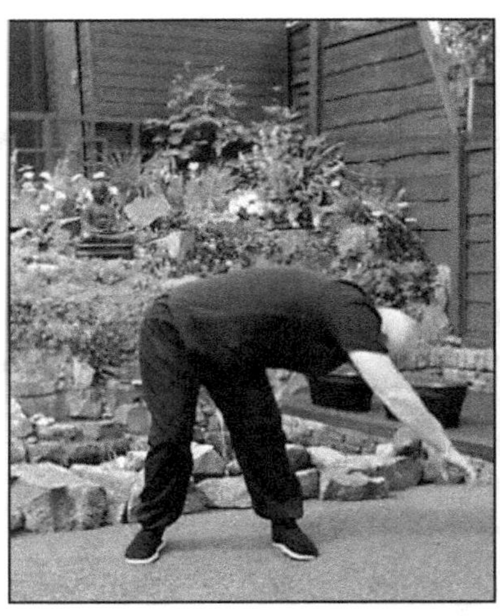
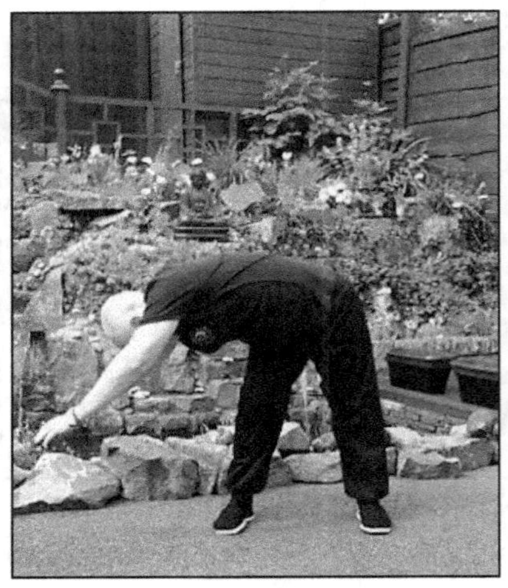

14. Support the Heavens

Stand with the feet shoulder-width apart in the basic *zhan zhuang* posture. Lift your palms upward, interlock the fingers and push the palms up to sky then sweep the arms out and down to the original position. If interlocking the fingers is painful, keep the palms separate.

When pushing upwards, there is a tendency to lose the root, which reduces the effectiveness of the posture. So, you should ensure when stretching upwards that you maintain the downward pull of the tailbone and root your heels/feet into the ground.

The stretch upwards should equal the stretch downwards. Finish in the basic *zhan zhuang* posture.

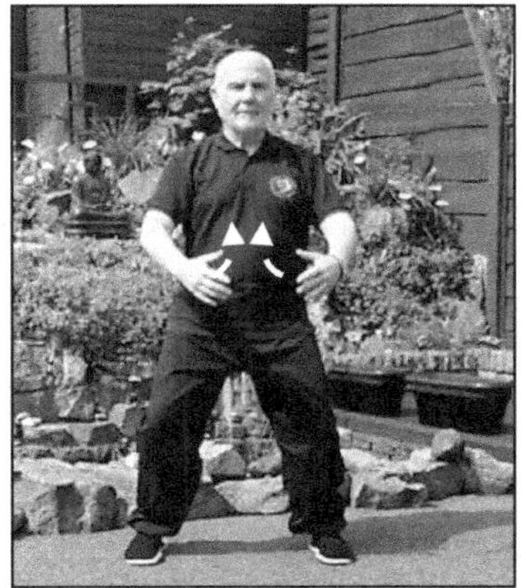

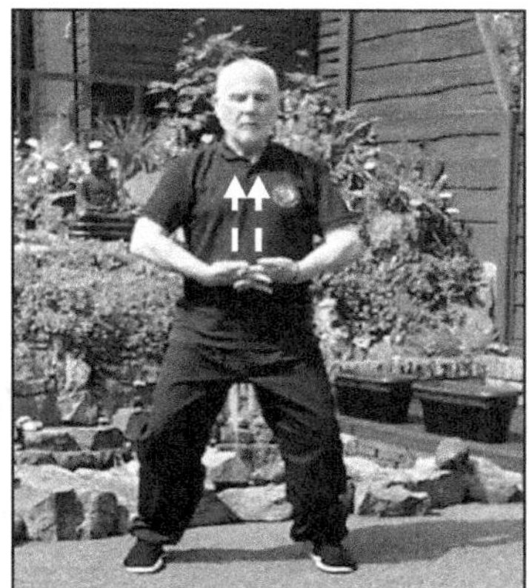

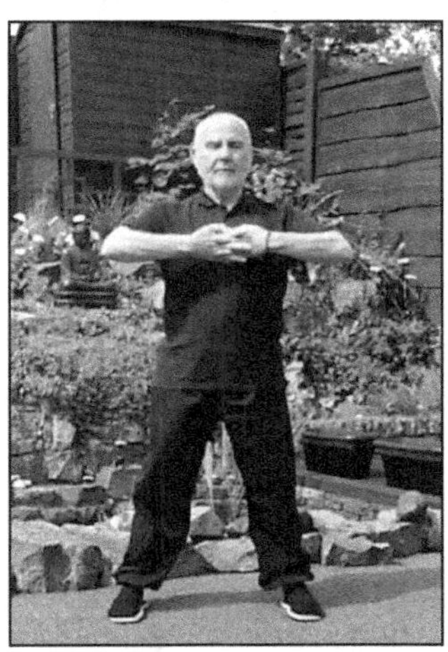

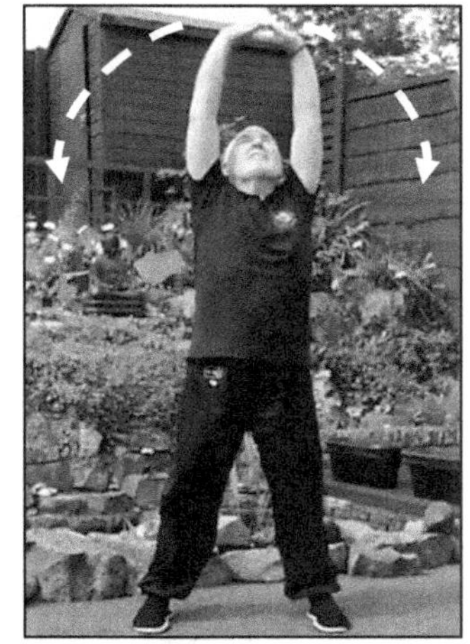

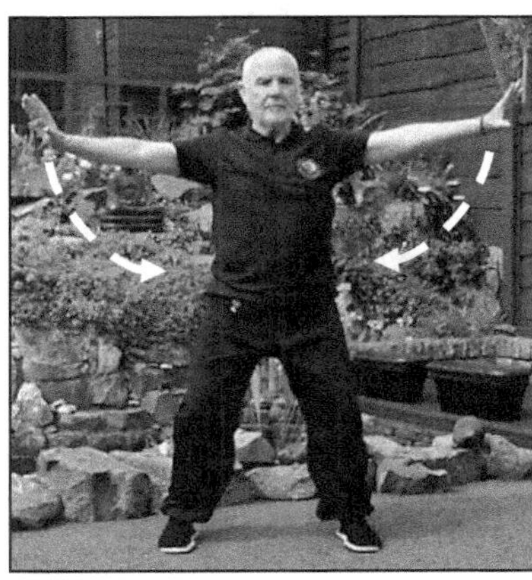

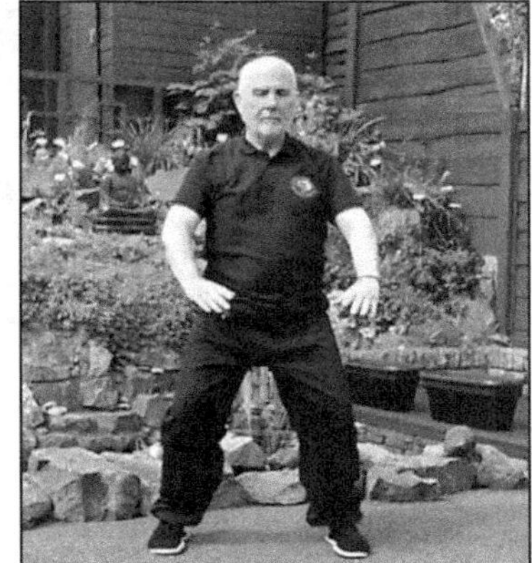

As with all the exercises, repeat a few times at first but gradually increase the repetitions as you become more capable. In addition, as you become stronger, hold the upward stretch for a short period. Remember, when you stretch up, straighten the legs a little and, with an opposing force to the hands, push down equally with the heels so that you do not lose your root. When you lower the arms, sink into the horse-riding posture, and relax the shoulders etc. For a more detailed explanation and version of this exercise, see Yang Jwing Ming (1990)

15. Rotate the Pelvis

There are several benefits to be derived from the following exercises. In Chi Gung theory, when this area is restricted, which is not uncommon due to injury, sedentary lifestyle, etc., the flow of Chi in important vessels is inhibited with a consequent adverse effect on health. This area is involved in major causes of back injury, pain, and restricted movement so we need to try to relax yet mobilise and strengthen the surrounding muscles and joints to improve Chi and blood flow, neural transmission, and structural support.

Stand with the feet shoulder-width apart in the basic posture. With hands on hips, gently rotate your pelvis clockwise, then anticlockwise.

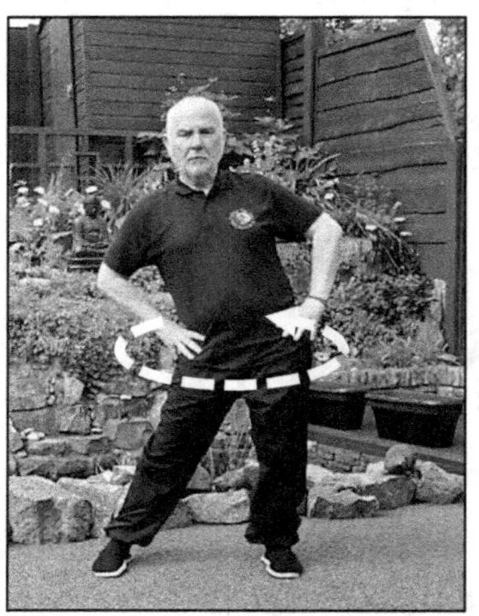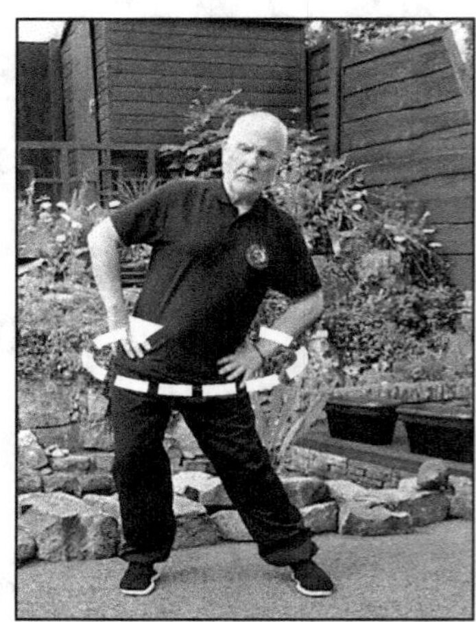

During backward rotation, there is a tendency to exaggerate the lumbar curve. To avoid this, try to push the low back out a little when rotating the pelvis backwards, as shown below.

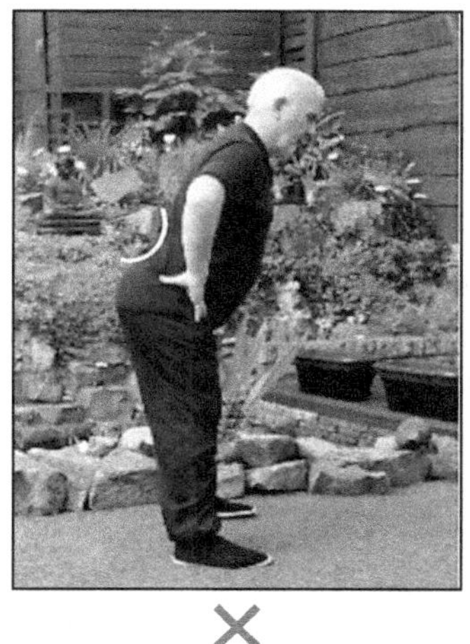 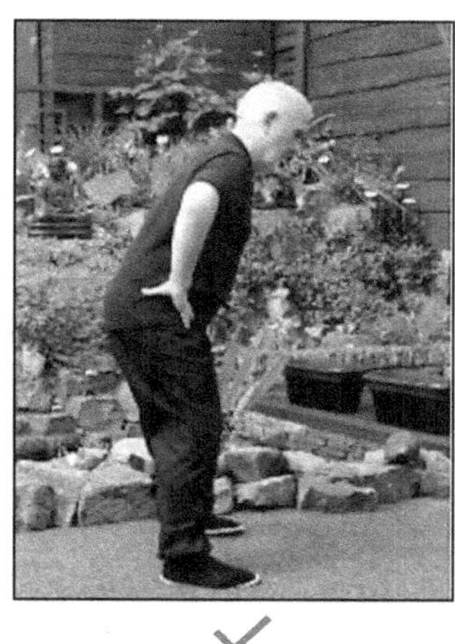

16. Knee Exercise 1 - Warm Up and Bend

Seated or standing, massage your knees, front, side and back and make sure to gently stimulate the tissues in and around the kneecaps. Then give the kneecaps a gentle wiggle. In addition, briskly rub all the muscles above and below the knee (avoid rubbing inflamed areas or varicose veins). This is usually sufficient to warm up the muscles, joints, ligaments, and tendons to help prevent injury.

Following on from the massage, stand with your feet together and gently bend and straighten the knees whilst still supporting them with the hands. Gradually, increase the angle of bend but keep it within the limits of comfort.

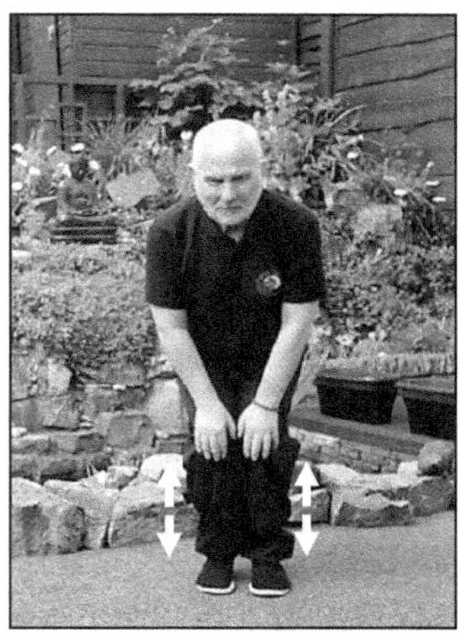

17. Knee exercise 2 - Rotate the Knees

If you practise sports or martial arts, a more extensive movement can be added. Place your hand on the knees and gently rotate them, first to the left a few times and then to the right. <u>Note</u> that this is not about bending your knees sideways *per se*. Of course, there will be some sideways movement, but it should not cause pain or injury. The aim is to ensure, within anatomical limitations, accessory movement - the capacity for some beneficial, additional play in the joint.

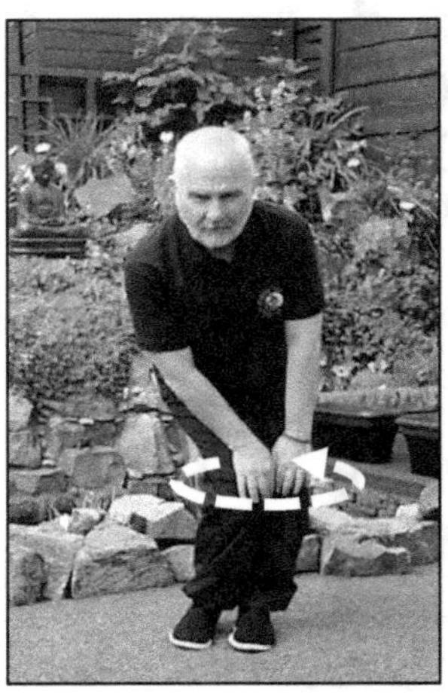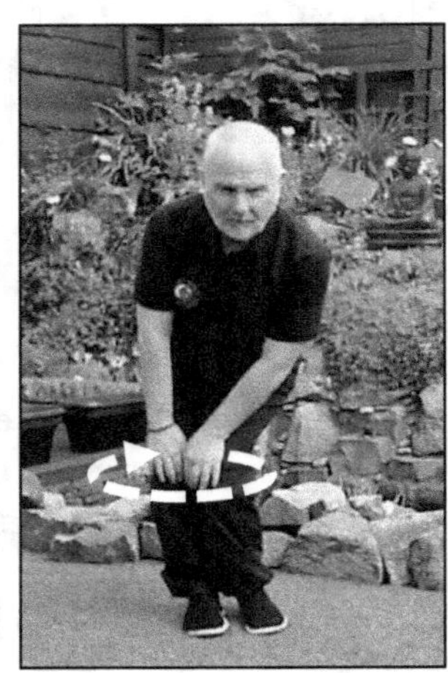

18. Side Leg Stretch

Stand in the basic posture with the feet shoulder-width apart and raise the crown of the head by gently tucking in the chin a little. Then, within your physical limitations and capability, step out to the left side a little more.

Shift your centre over to the left and hold the stretch for a few seconds. Keep your bottom in and avoid twisting the body.

Make sure the weight bearing knee is above the foot and avoid twisting and distorting the knee joint. You can make some adjustment with foot position to avoid knee strain, e.g., the weighted foot angled outward. Repeat a few times on each side.

When shifting from one side to the other, try to avoid "drifting" across. You should move with purpose and muscular control of both knee joints.

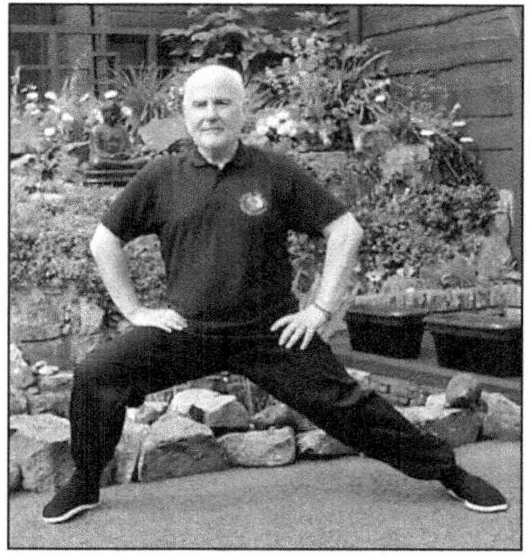 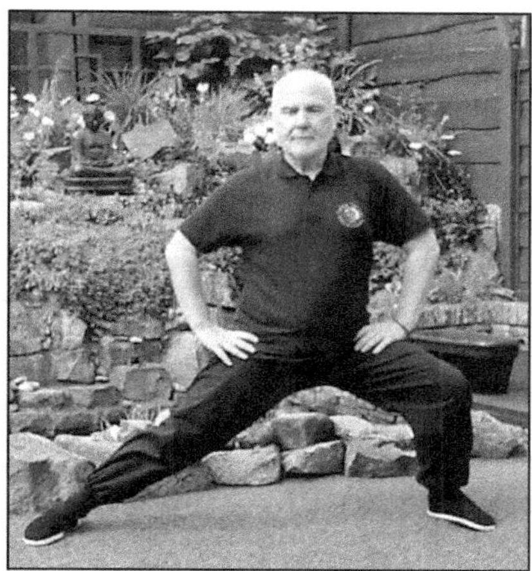

19. Lunge Stretch

Return to the basic position, i.e., stand with the feet shoulder-width apart in the basic posture and raise the crown of the head by gently tucking in the chin a little. Then, within your limitations, step out to the left side a little more but adjusting the weight bearing foot to point to the left side. Lunge and hold for a few seconds. Keep your bottom tucked in, avoid twisting the body and make sure the weight bearing knee is above the foot to prevent undue torsion. Repeat on both sides.

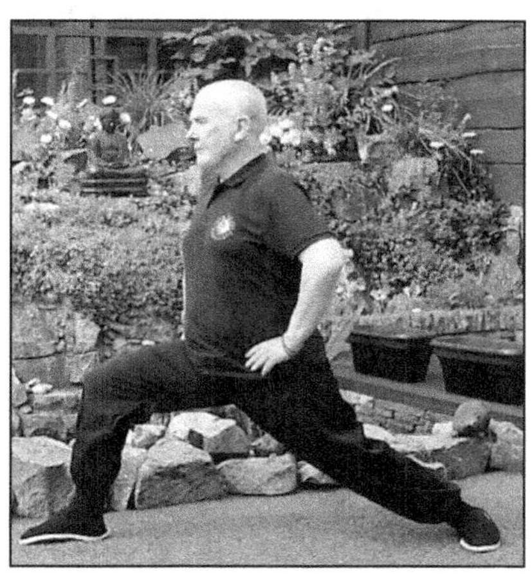 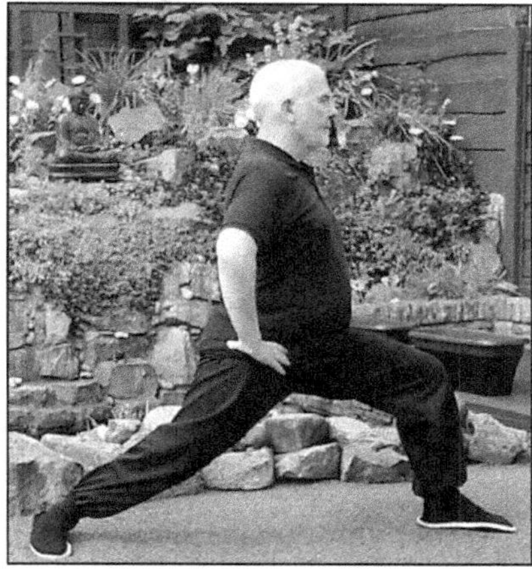

20. Hamstring and Calf Stretch

Although this exercise incorporates strengthening, stretching, and twisting of the spine, it is important not to emphasise the spinal stretch too much. Instead, you should focus just on the feeling of stretching the back of the leg. Once you feel that stretch, stop bending and try to mentally relax the muscles for a few moments.

Return to the basic position, i.e., stand with the feet shoulder-width apart in the basic posture, raise the crown of the head by gently tucking in the chin a little. Place your hands on the hips and turn the left foot on the heel to point up to the left at about 45 degrees. Gently and carefully rotate the right shoulder toward the left knee.

Do not attempt to go beyond your safety limit. Remember, once you feel the stretch in the back of your leg hold it for a few seconds but try to relax the muscles. Avoid undue twisting and distortion of the weight-bearing knee joint. Repeat on both sides.

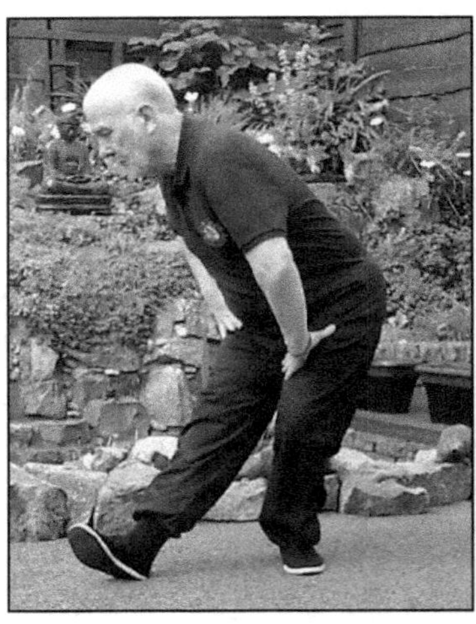 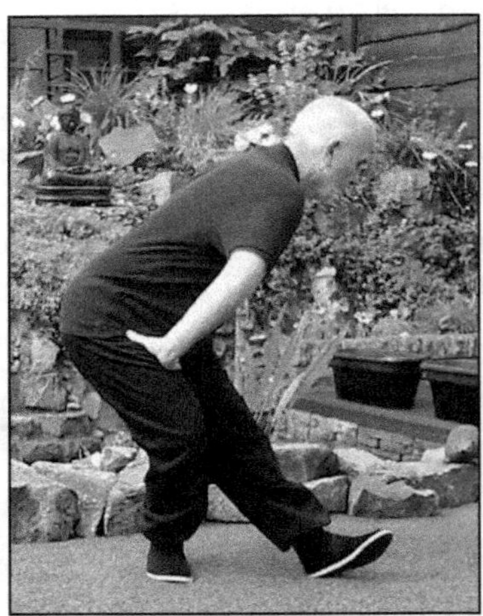

21. Ankle Rotation

Return to basic position, i.e., stand with the feet shoulder-width apart in the basic posture and raise the crown of the head by gently tucking in the chin a little. The primary aim of this exercise is to encourage mobility and accessory movement in the ankle. However, it is also useful in encouraging knee and hip health and mobility.

Place one foot slightly to the rear of the weight bearing foot (using the tip of your shoe as a pivot) and rock the heel from side to side until you feel the ankle, knee and hip are moving loosely, then rotate the heel clockwise a few times and then anticlockwise. If you are doing this effectively the ankle, knee and hip movement should feel very loose and floppy. Repeat on both legs.

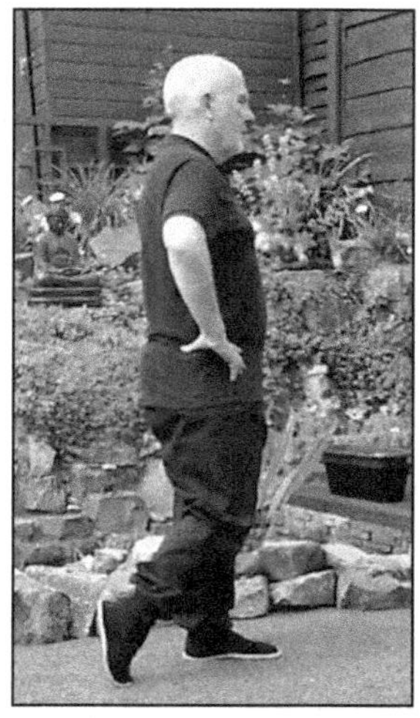

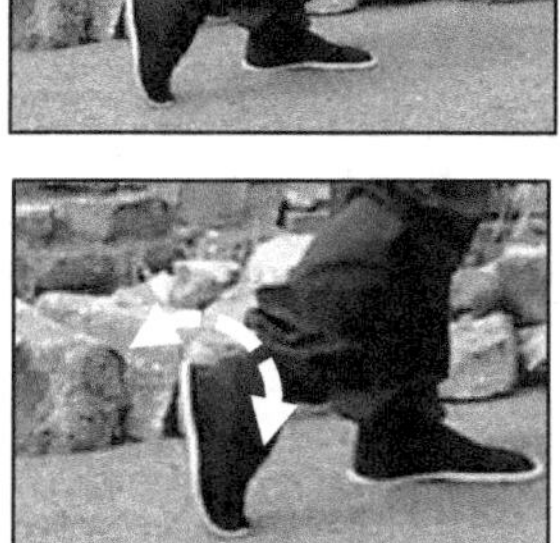

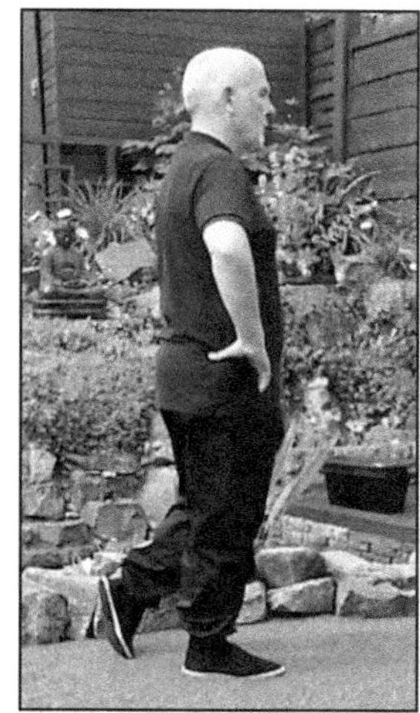

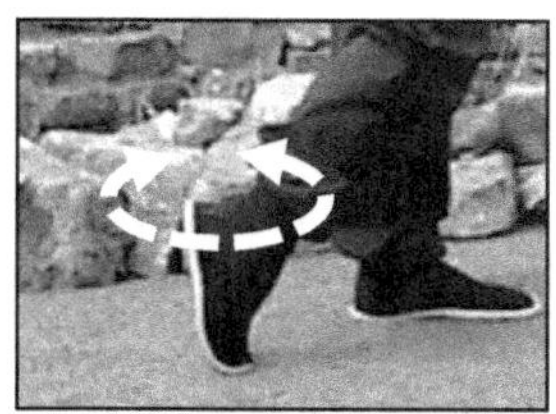

Unless you have excellent balance and control when standing on one leg, you should hold on to something when doing this exercise. Otherwise, you will be unable to allow the rocking leg and joints to become fully relaxed and flaccid.

✱✱✱✱✱✱✱✱✱✱✱✱✱✱✱✱✱✱✱✱✱✱✱

The latter exercises are stand-alone, i.e., they can be practised without any other exercises as an effective, regular, daily routine. (Note the words "regular" and "daily", sporadic will not do it!). However, by means of extension one can incorporate slowing down, meditative exercise, while continuing to develop mobility, flexibility, and strength. Any Chi Gung form can be incorporated but I find the following set to be popular and useful for most people and most conditions.

4 SLOWING DOWN EXERCISES – CHI GUNG

What is Chi Gung?

The Neijing, an ancient Chinese medical classic, states:

"In ancient times people lived according to natural ways… Thus, they formulated practices such as Dao-in, an exercise combining stretching, massaging, and breathing to promote energy flow, and meditation to help harmonise themselves with the universe."*

Because the balance and efficient flow of energy or *Chi* is perhaps the essential aspect of "natural ways" in the Chinese theory of health, such methods can be collectively referred to as Chi Gung* (working with Chi). Therefore, the practice of Chi Gung, when working with Chi, utilises a variety of methods to maintain the health and well-being of individuals, such as the gentle rhythmic exercises of *Tai Chi* and *Eight Pieces of Brocade* (*Baduanjin*), or the more power-oriented *Iron Thread Form* (*Tid Sid Kuen*), etc. The form studied here, adapted from a more modern synthesis (e.g., of Tai Chi, Chi Gung and perhaps *Dao-in**) originally developed by Lin Hou Sheng (www.linhousheng.com), is commonly known as *Tai Chi-Chi Gung* or *18 Postures* (*Shibashi*).

How Does Chi Gung Exercise Work?

The slow, condensing and expanding movements of Chi Gung contract, stretch, stimulate, and relax the muscles and soft tissues of the body, and help to increase bone density and joint mobility. When combined with specific breathing techniques, Chi Gung improves respiration, circulation, and lymph movement, thus nourishing tissues and aiding the removal of unwanted substances from the body. More importantly, within Chinese medical theory, its postures and breathing techniques enhance and regulate the flow of Chi or energy throughout the body and generate a field of energy known as "Guardian Chi" that helps protect one from pathological environmental changes.

Distinctively, Chi Gung and Tai Chi employ positive mental intention, so such exercises are sometimes termed "meditation in action". This meditative aspect of Chi Gung, coordinated with its rhythmic postures, engenders clarity of mind, calms the emotions, and invigorates the spirit. Thus, Chi Gung helps create a healthy, coordinated mind and body better able to deal with the pathogenic stressors that individuals may encounter in their daily lives.

Chi Gung Stationary form

In the chronology of Chi Gung development, the following sequence is a relatively new and more populist form of Chi Gung. It is useful because it does not necessarily require a knowledge of, or belief in, the more esoteric concepts that are associated with Chi Gung. Yet, it incorporates its meditative physical exercise and breathing methods to beneficial effects. Because of this, it is useful as a stand-alone exercise or as a basic training method for its more dynamic relative, Tai Chi Chuan (*Taijiquan*). So, I have presented this form here because of its suitability for both purposes. However, as a personal choice of enhancement based on experience, I have offered some adaptations, which incorporate a flavour of my own favoured systems of Gung Fu, i.e., *Xing Yi*, *Ba Gua* and *Hung Kuen*, which I have found to provide more effective postural stance/alignment, strengthening and flexibility. Each posture should be repeated, e.g., 3, 6 or 9 times each.

** Technically, Dao-in is a form of yoga, but then one could argue that so is Chi Gung, in which case, one could argue that so is Tai Chi. A simple compromise might be to say that Chi Gung is a more dynamic form of Dao-in and Tai Chi is a more dynamic form of Chi Gung.*

Posture 1. Regulating the Breath

This posture is found, in some form, in every Chi Gung sequence. It encourages physical and mental relaxation and grounding, and regulates natural breathing, i.e., appropriate to energetic requirements of any given posture (It has other connotations with regard the Taoist alchemical transformation and movement of Chi but that requires a relatively complicated visualisation, to be practised only under the guidance of a teacher and at more spiritual levels by an adept). Begin in *Wu chi* posture with a "cleansing" breath then step out to basic posture 1. Breathe-in naturally as you raise the arms and breath-out as you lower them.

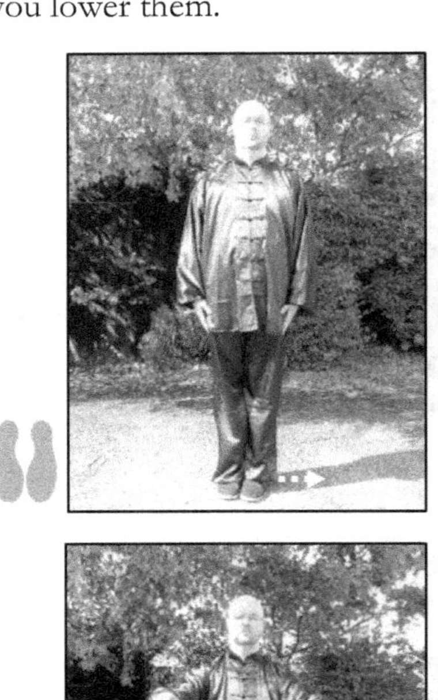
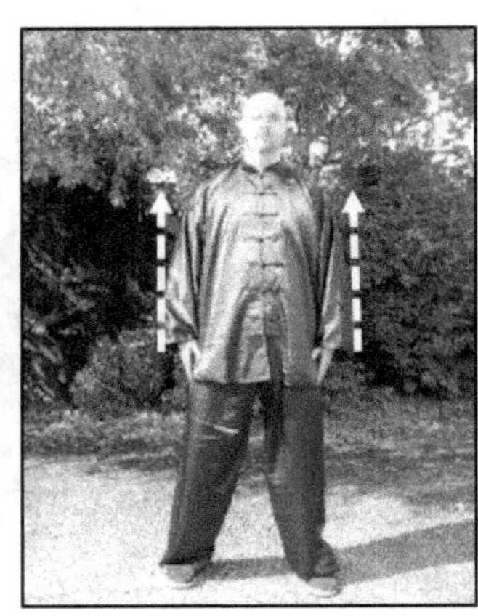
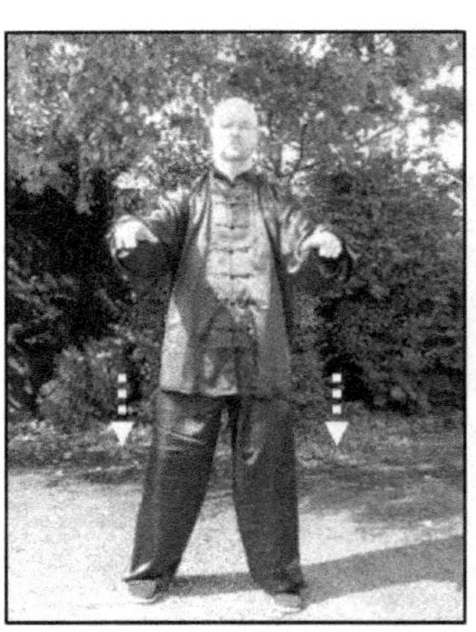
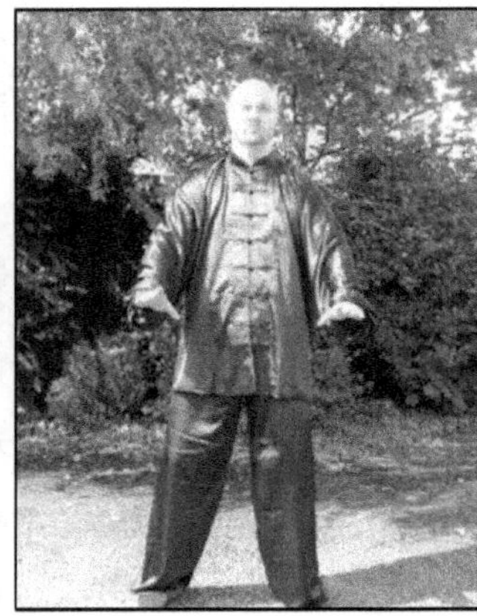

The hands describe an upward, forward arc and a downward, inward arc. Repeat the arm movements several times but with each flowing up and down movement of the palms, coordinate straightening and bending of the knees respectively. Ensure knee and foot alignment.

Posture 2. Opening the Chest

Flowing through from the previous posture, this movement is similar but more expansive.

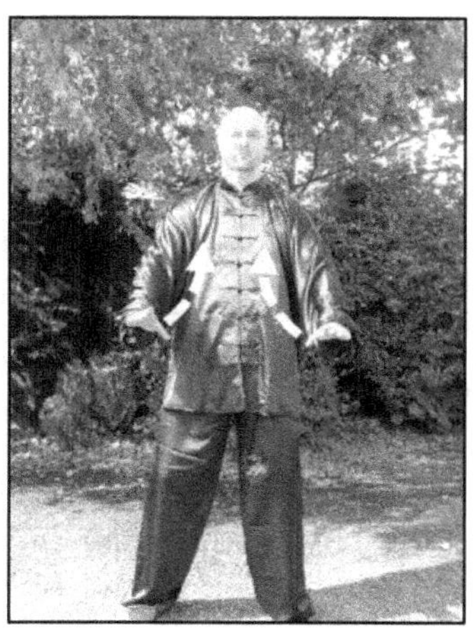
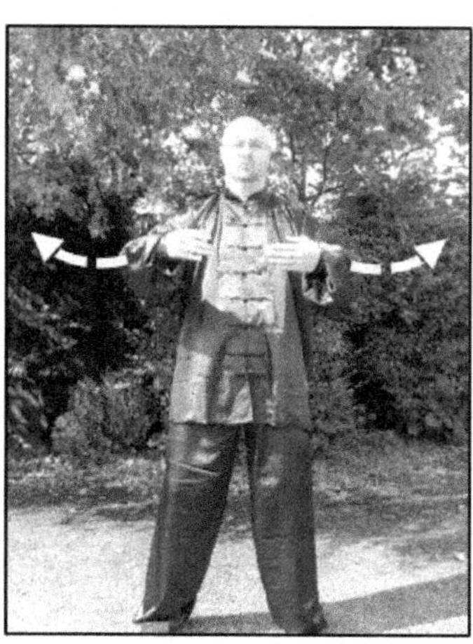
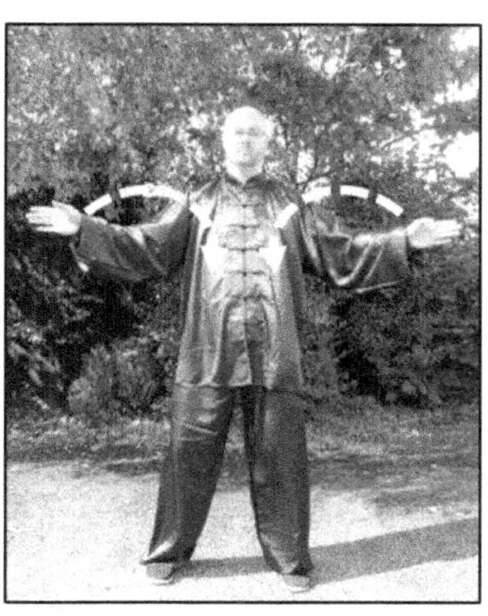
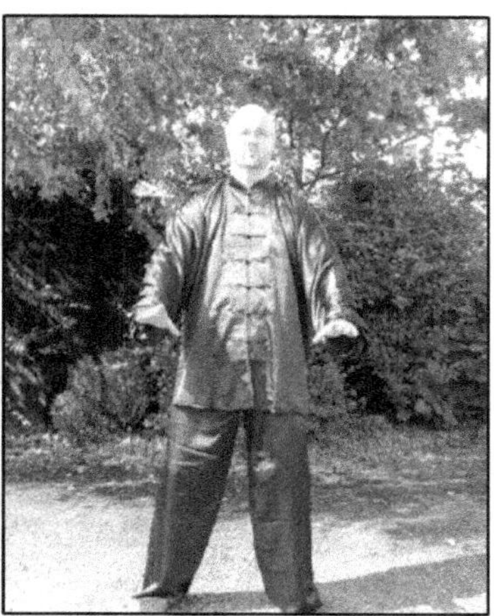

It is helpful to visualise a balloon pushing the palms up and expanding to push them apart. Then, you compress the balloon, pushing out the air to gently press it down to the resting position. As with the previous posture, coordinate the raising and lowering of the palms with straightening and bending the knees respectively.

Posture 3. Dancing with the Rainbow

Visualise opening a rainbow above your head, sinking into the horse-riding posture. Now, shift your weight to the right leg and step out with the left foot on the diagonal in a resting or "empty posture".

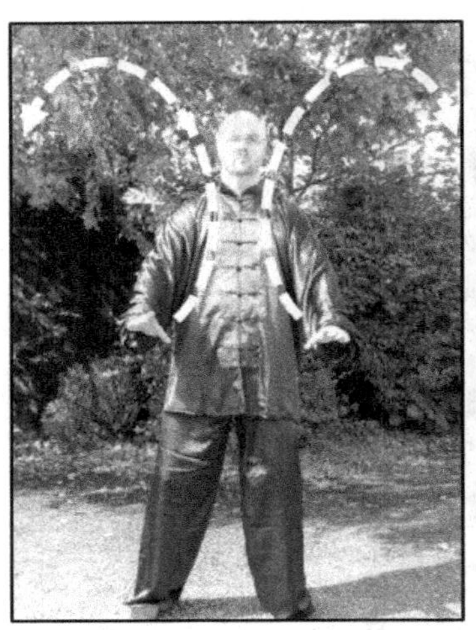

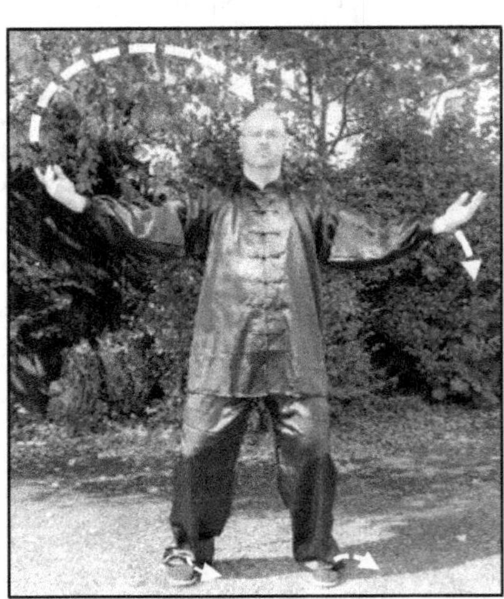

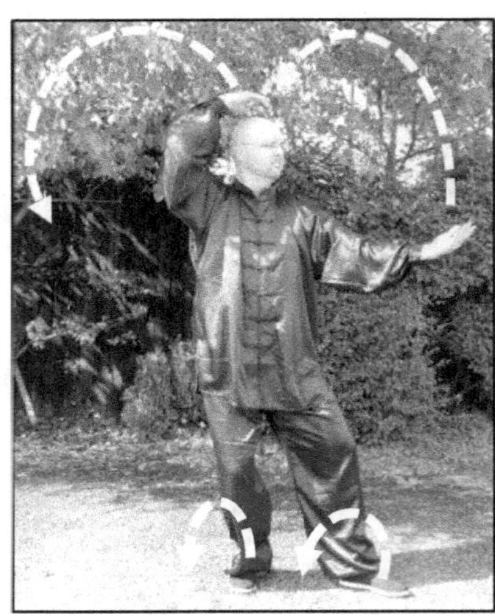

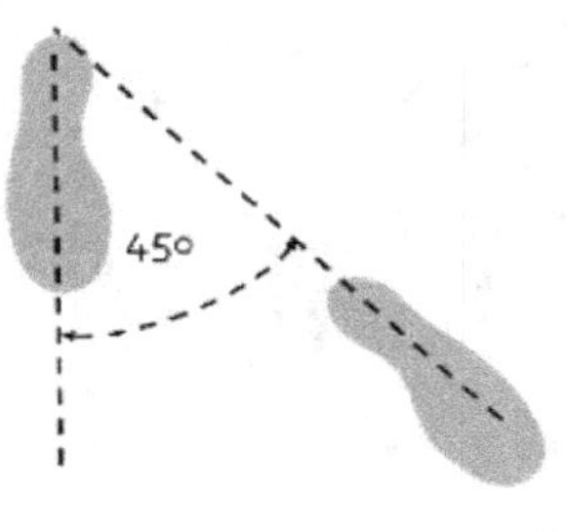

In Yang style, from which this form is partly developed, this stance is a back-sitting posture, and the weight distribution is commonly 60%

on the back leg and 40% on the front. You can use this or a slightly more even distribution of weight, but, as much as possible, we want to try and develop stronger, single leg rooting and stability within movement. Providing that you do not have knee problems, you can take up the Xing Yi stance of *San Ti Shi*, i.e., up to 100% on the rear and almost 0% on the front (80:20 or 60:40 for beginners). Ensure your bent knees are aligned with your feet and that you maintain the correct spinal/pelvic posture (avoid allowing the weight bearing hip to push outwards and become misaligned). At the same time as you step, raise the right hand above the head and lower the left slightly.

Following on, step back with the left foot and then step diagonally with the right. With a flowing motion complete the hand posture to the right side. The hands move as per the direction of the arrows in the diagrams. Repeat a few or several times each side. Remember to keep the shoulders relaxed and sink the pelvis.

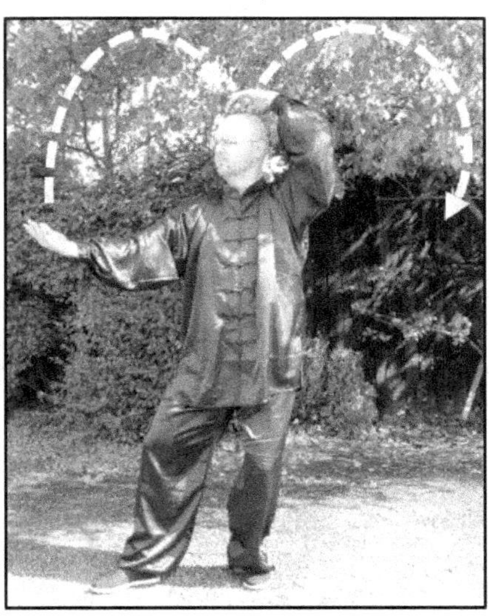

Posture 4. Separating the Clouds

Step back into the horse-riding posture. Whilst maintaining the correct spinal posture, sink a little more and bend forward as you cross the hands in front. Continue to sweep the arms across and upwards to cross above the head or as high as you can. Sweep them out in an arc and repeat. As a general rule in Chi Gung, you should <u>stretch</u> upwards but <u>relax</u> downwards. Repeat the desired number of times.

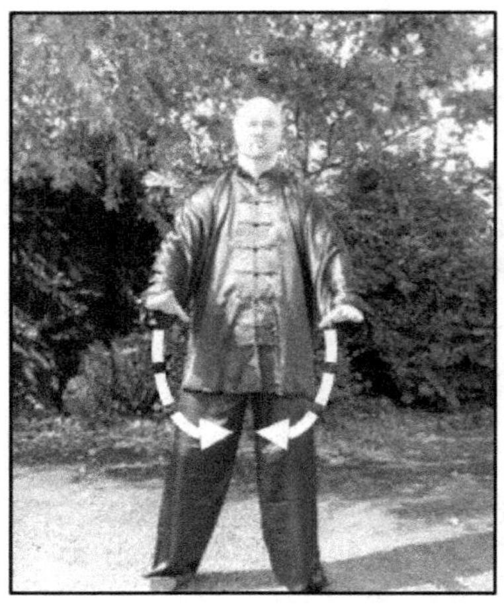
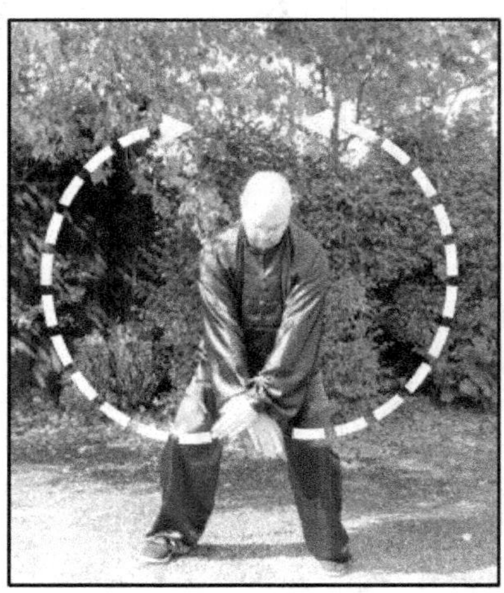

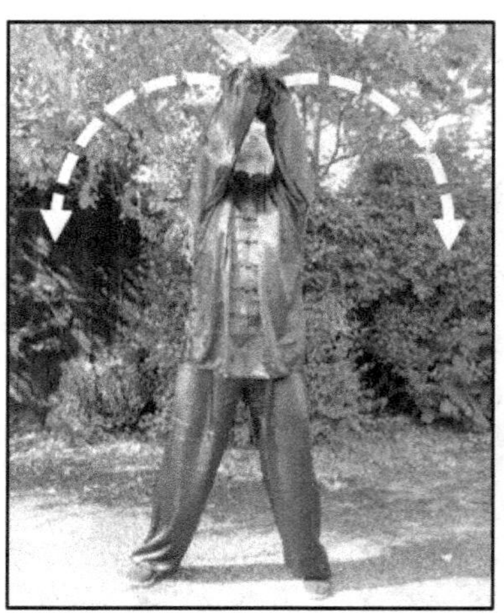
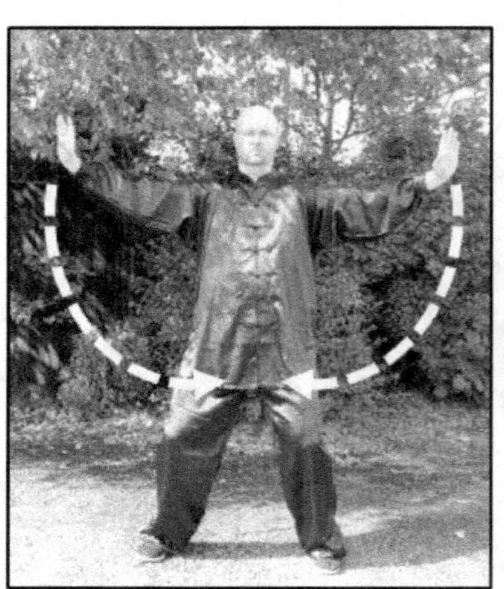

The picture on the right demonstrates this posture in the classic *Hung Kuen* horse-riding posture.

This lower stance is useful for developing strong root, balance and proprioception but should not be practised if one has a knee injury or without appropriate instruction.

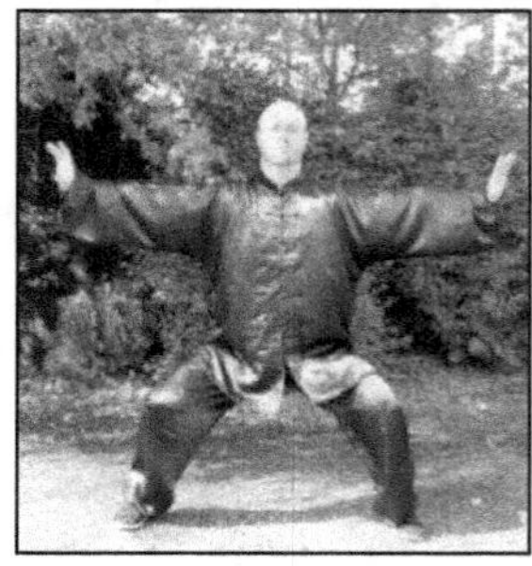

Posture 5. Reverse Reeling Arms

Although adapted from the moving posture of Tai Chi called *Step Backwards to Repulse the Monkey (Dao Nien Hou)*, this movement is performed here in a strong horse-riding posture. The arms rotate in a smooth, flowing, and relaxed manner, a little like the freestyle swimming motion. From the basic posture, lift both hands with the palms upward - the left hand to the front and the right hand to the side, then pull down the left hand along your centreline and push the right forward. Avoid undue raising of the shoulders and elbows. Repeat on both sides.

Once familiar with the movement you can coordinate a loose and relaxed waist movement as shown in the diagram below.

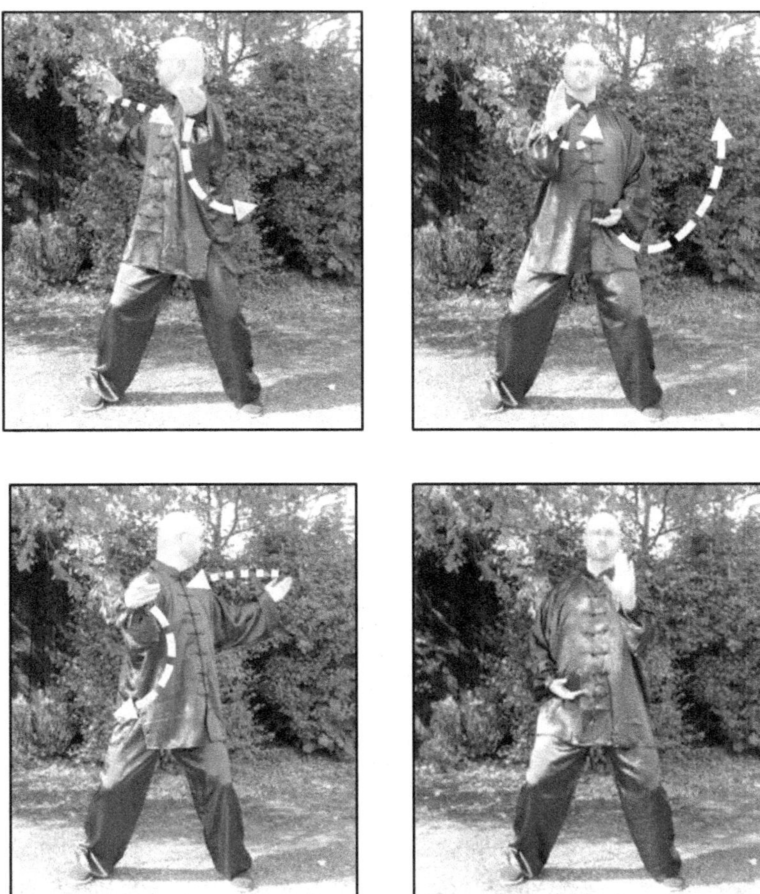

There is a tendency for the body to find the easiest way to do things and therefore, in this case, to twist the knees and bend the low back in an effort to make a large turn of the waist. To avoid this, try to keep the natural spinal curve and a strong stance for optimum benefit with regard to developing flexibility, root strength, stability and improved proprioception.

Posture 6. Rowing the Boat in the Centre of the Lake
Continuing from the previous posture, perform a rowing-like movement by sweeping both arms in an arc, outwards, backward, and upward to then make a light fist at the shoulders. Then, as you sink into a lower horse stance, push the fists forward and down (like rowing a boat), opening the fists into the Tai Chi palm. Once again sweep the arms back up as you rise ready to repeat the movement or brush down to finish.

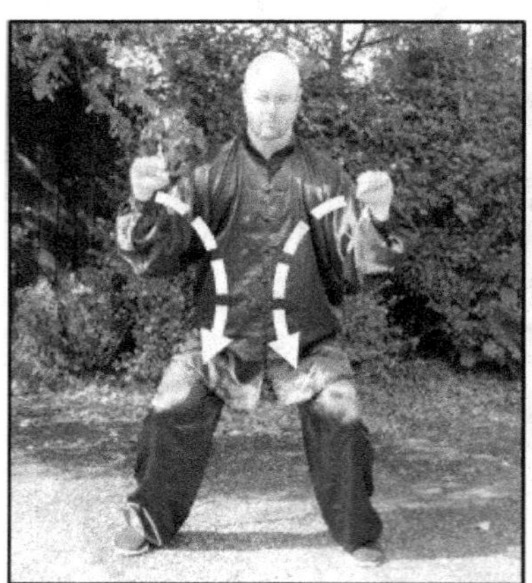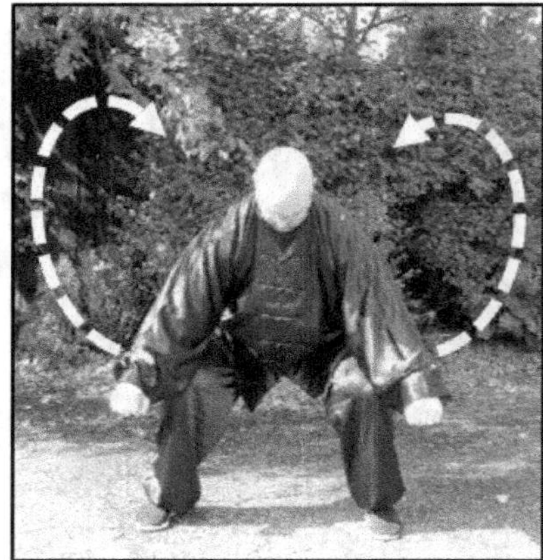

Posture 7. Supporting the Ball in Front of the Chest/Shoulder
Continuing from the previous posture, visualise catching a ball in front of the *dantien* and raising it across the body, one side then the other. You should sink into the horse-riding posture, then raise the right palm-up to the left side, at the same time raising the right heel.

Stretch out when turning to the side but then relax when sinking into the horse-riding posture and lowering the heel. Keep the waist loose and relaxed. Remember to alternate from side to side in a balanced and flowing manner. Repeat an equal number of times left and right.

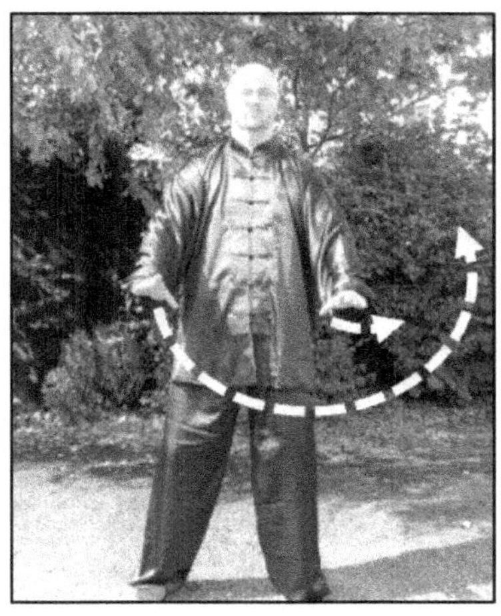 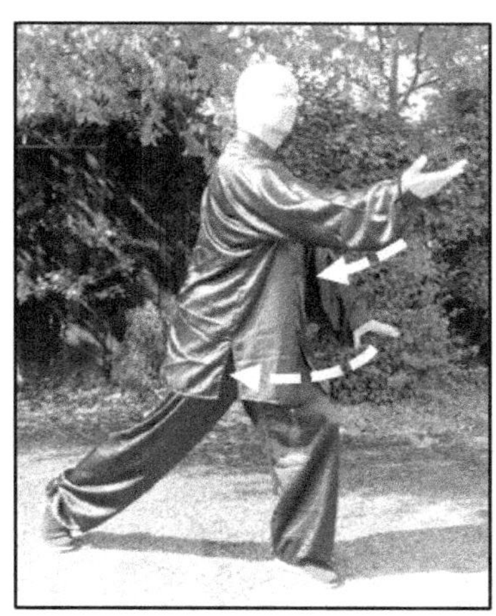

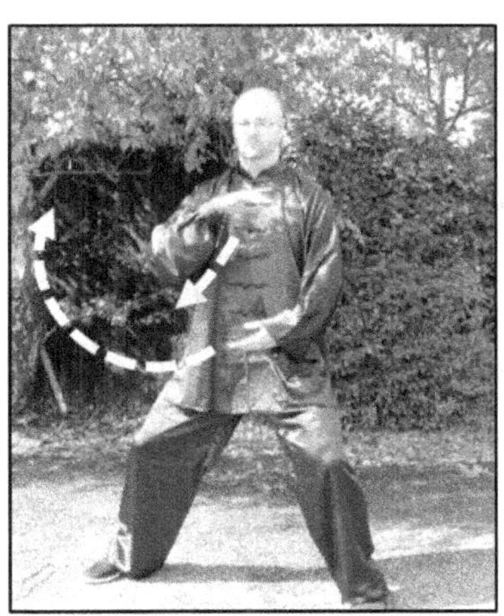 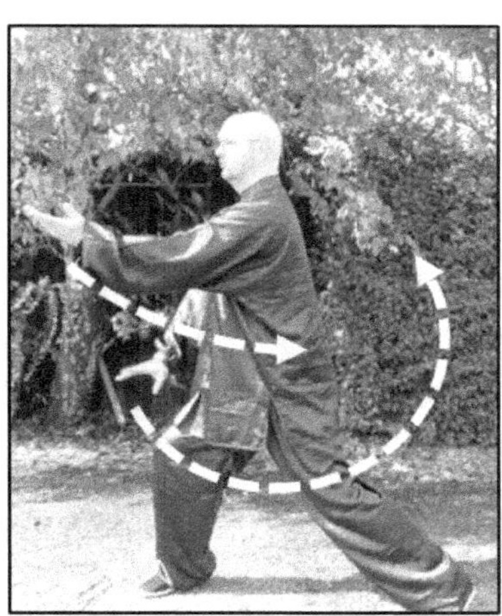

Posture 8. Turn the Body to Gaze at the Moon

Continue from the previous posture but now visualise holding the ball (moon) in both hands raising it across the body - one side then the other. If capable, turn to gaze up between the hands. Take care not to overstretch at first as this might strain the rib muscles. When you become more flexible you can begin to turn slightly to the rear.

As you turn to stetch and gaze up, at the same time raise the right heel. Keep the waist loose and relaxed. Remember to alternate from side to side in a balanced and flowing manner.

Repeat an equal number of times left and right.

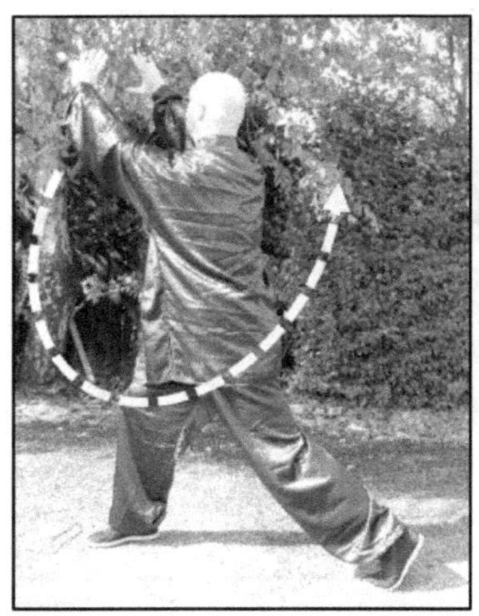 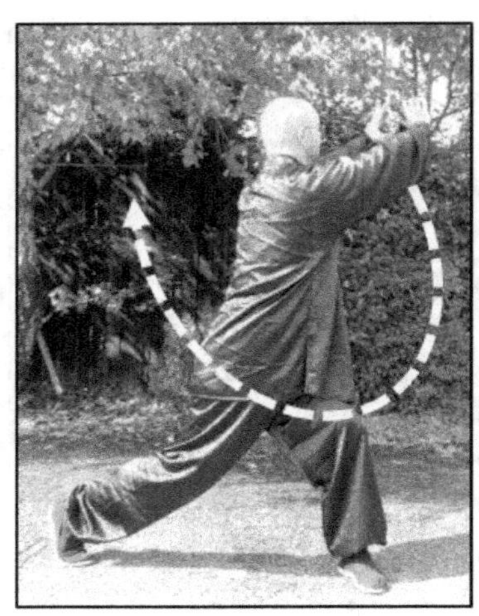

Posture 9. Turning Waist and Pushing Palm

Stand in the horse-riding posture (Tai Chi or Hung Kuen style, depending on capability) and draw the hands in to make a fist just above the hips. Establish a strong root and try to avoid weakening it by twisting the knees and thighs. Open the right fist into a splayed palm and push forward and slightly upwards. Without allowing the palm to drift, turn your body to the right and then turn the head further to look behind. Now, relax and pull the left hand back to make a fist just above the hip then push the right palm forward and turn the body and head to the left. Again, your body will try to find the easiest way to do this by twisting the thigh and flexing the lumbar spine, avoid this.

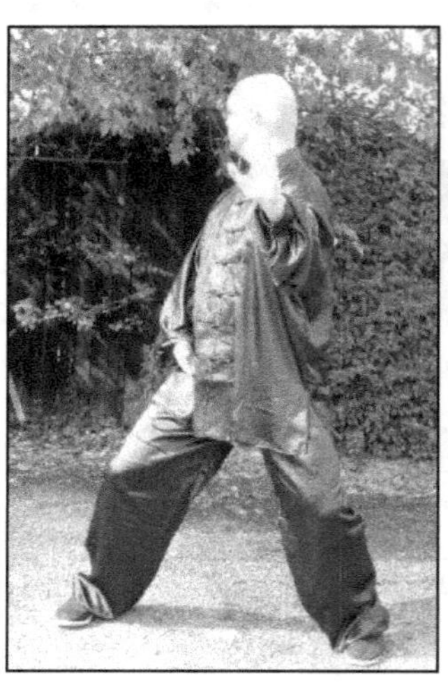 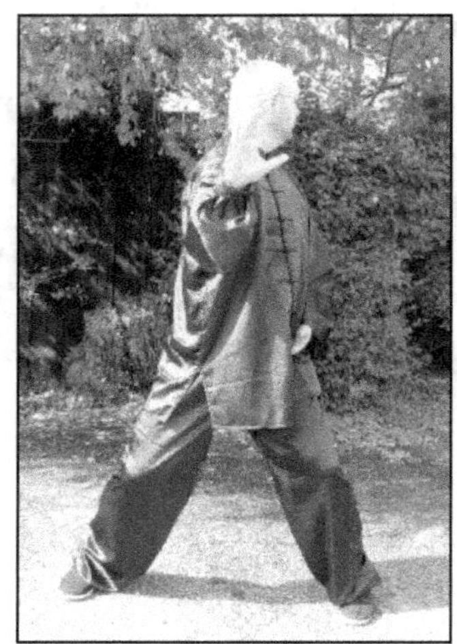

Posture 10. Hands Drifting in the Clouds

Following on from the previous posture, swirl the left palm across the front-lower-body and upwards, then continue swirling the palm backwards across the front-upper-body. The shoulder girdle, wrist and elbow should remain relaxed. Then make a similar circle on the right. Then practise to coordinate the hand movements on both sides. The left arm and hand rotate anti-clockwise, the right rotate clockwise. You should also try to incorporate a relaxed waist movement from side to side.

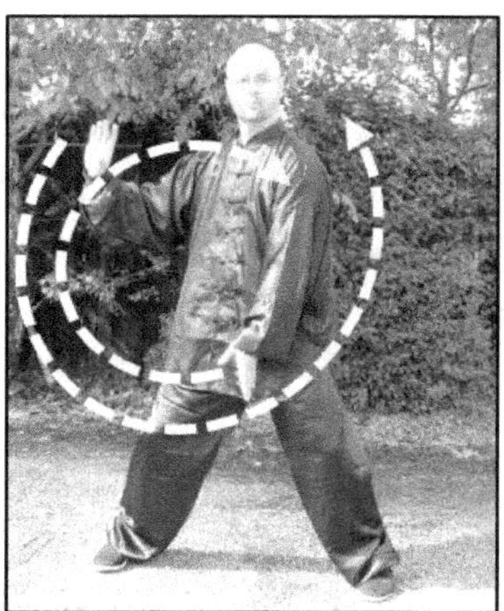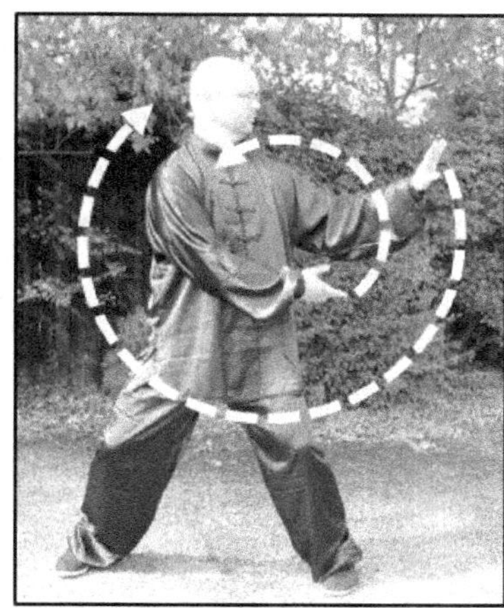

Initially, until you get used to the movement and are more able to coordinate the alternating palms, it might be helpful to practise this posture one side at a time, i.e., circle the left palm anticlockwise, then circle the right palm clockwise.

Posture 10a - Advanced alternative: Bagua Palm Change

This posture is more extensive than cloud hands and is adapted from the internal art of *Baguazhang*. It requires a quite complicated and coordinated twisting movement of the palms, body, and spine. The movement develops greater coordination, root stability and more sensitive balance and proprioception, which are essential for the sudden and often spontaneous changes of direction and pace associated with *Bagua*.

To commence, both hands drive upwards at the centre of the body, palms twisting inwards, the left is outermost and the right innermost.

Continue to drive the palms upward and then outward and downward in an arc, toward the left side/rear. At the same time, twist your waist to the left side/rear. Now, the left-hand twists inward and the right hand outward to perform a similar arcing movement toward the right/rear. Alternate left and right in a very smooth and flowing circular pattern… I said it was complicated!

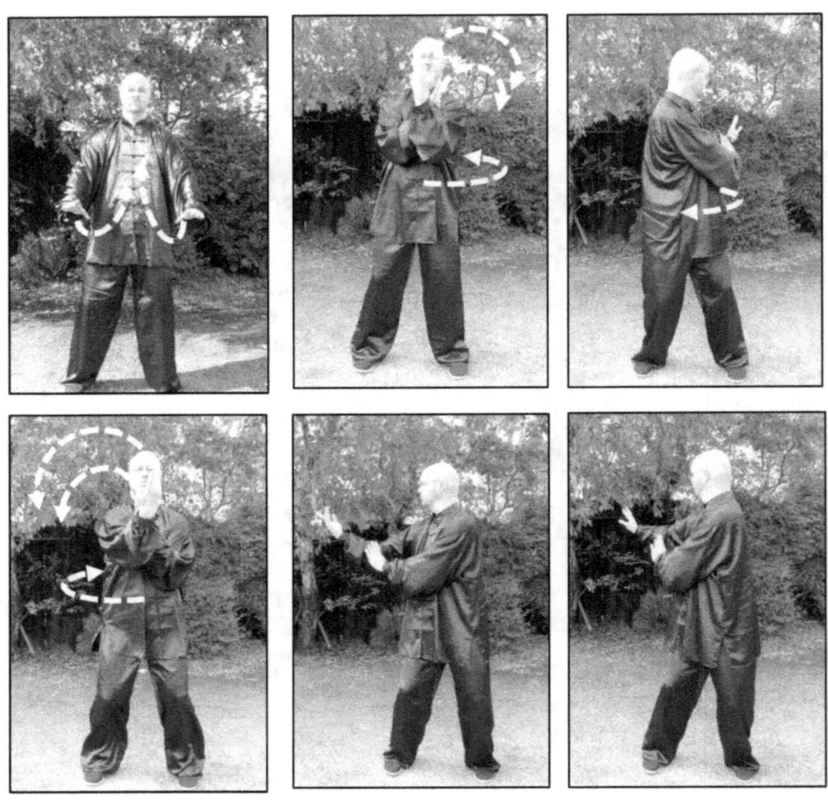

When proficient and able, you can then incorporate stepping into this posture. Initially, the stance should be relatively high but eventually you might be able to lower the posture, which will help develop more strength in the lower limbs. However, the essential training here, as mentioned previously, is to develop greater coordination, root stability and more sensitive proprioception. Stepping is shown below.

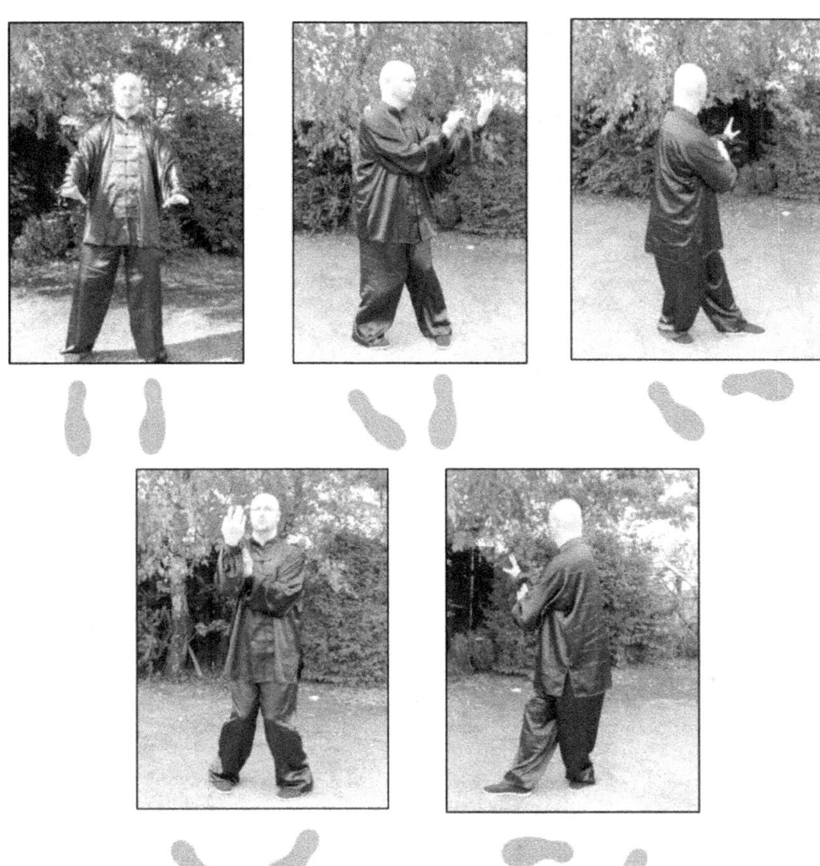

Posture 11. Dredging the Sea and Looking at the Sky

Following on from the previous posture, purposefully, but slowly and gently, step out with the left foot on the diagonal. Shift into a forward bow posture (70% on the front leg, 30% on the rear). Carry out similar but more extensive hand movements to Posture 3 *Separating the Clouds*. As you shift forward, relax the whole of the spine, using the left thigh to help support the body.

In addition to the general function of these exercises, this posture enables comfortable stretching and relaxation of the vertebral muscles and joints. This being the case, you should, at first, avoid excessive bending until the muscles develop some degree of strength and flexibility.

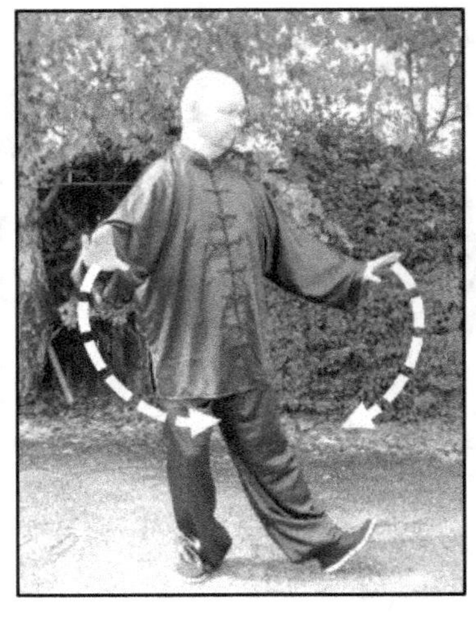 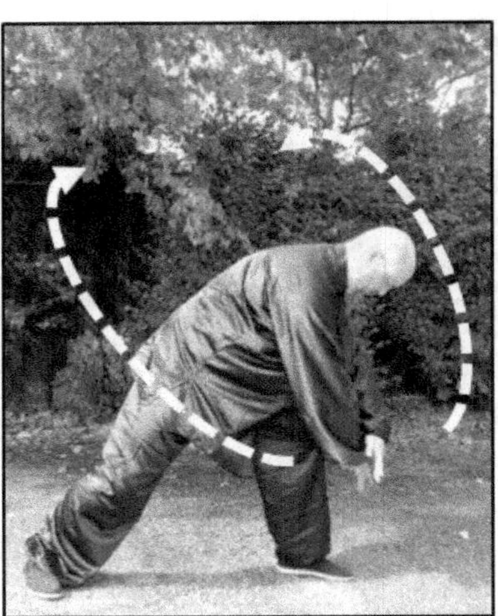

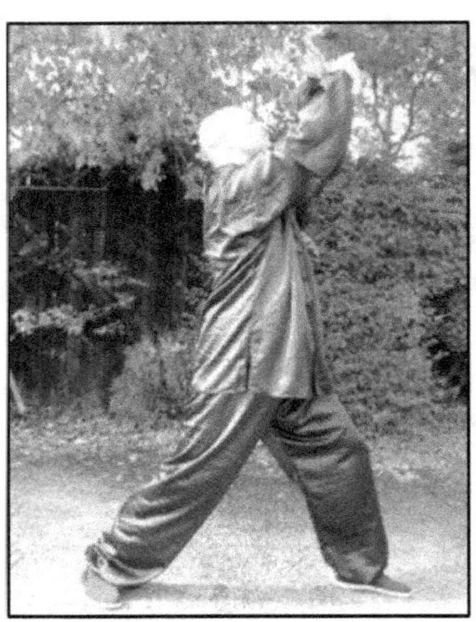 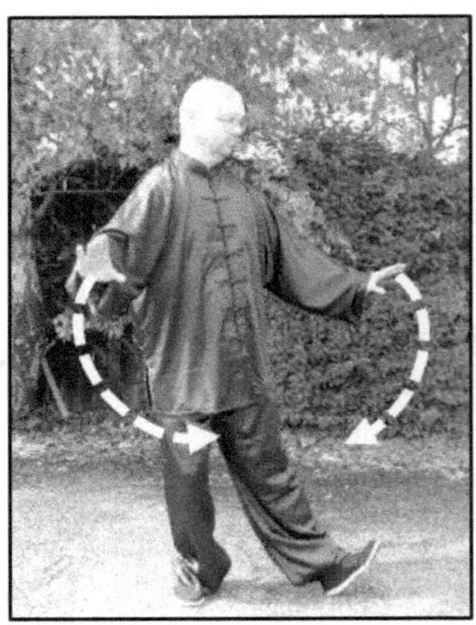

As you rise, support the lumbar spine by first shifting your weight back onto the rear leg and pushing up from the rear foot as you rock back into a resting posture or *San Ti Shi*. To complete the movement, stretch the arms upwards and outwards like separating clouds.

Take care not to overstretch or rise suddenly from the stooping position. Be sure to sit backwards and curl the spine up using the energy from your rooted foot.

Following an appropriate number of movements on the left side, step back and repeat on the right side.

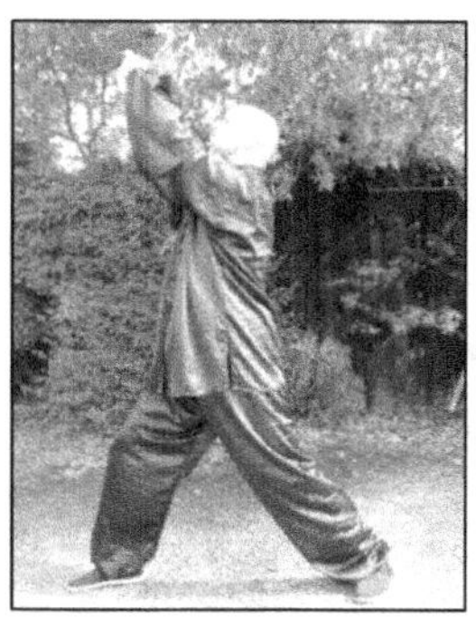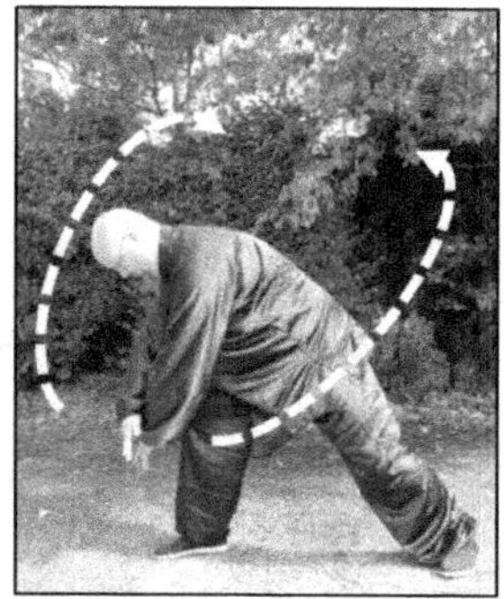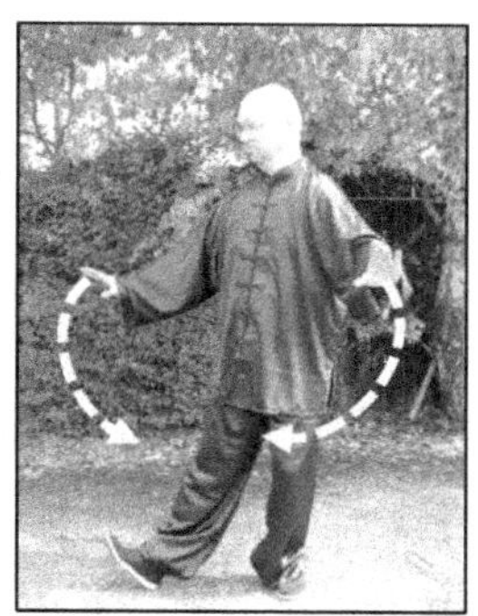

Posture 12. Pushing the Waves

In this posture you need to use a little more visualisation. From the previous posture, step out on the left diagonal and sweep your arms up as though you were catching the crest of a big wave coming toward you.

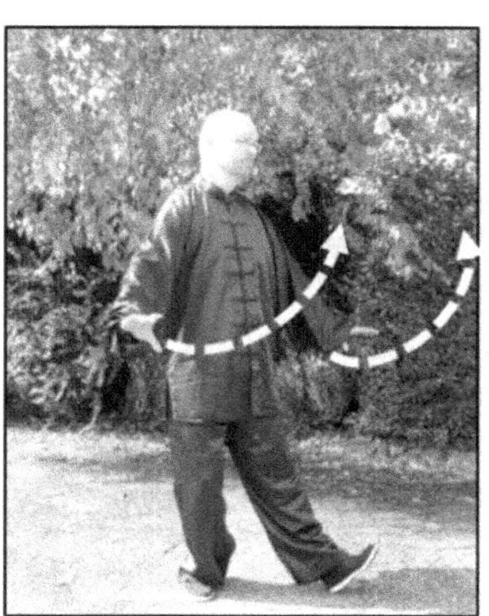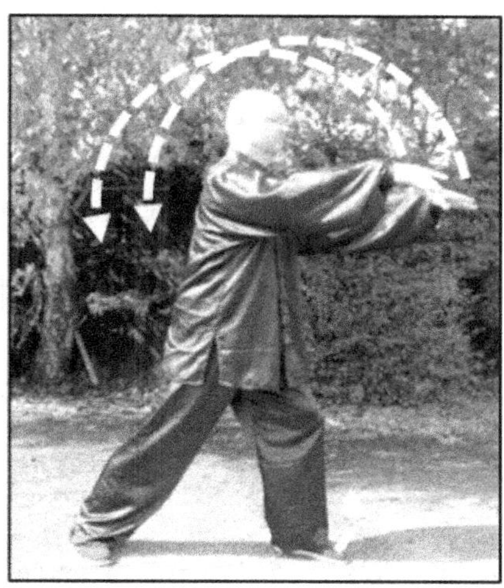

Go with the flow of the wave by riding it back and then when its energy is guided down into your root, use this stored energy to push the water back out to sea. As you rock back onto the right foot lift the toes of the left foot and stretch the left leg. In the original form the rear heel is raised on the forward movement, but I find it is best, for Chi Gung purposes, to keep the heel on the floor. Weight distribution on the forward movement should be 70% on the front leg and 30%

on the rear; the backward movement depends on your limitations as in Posture 3.

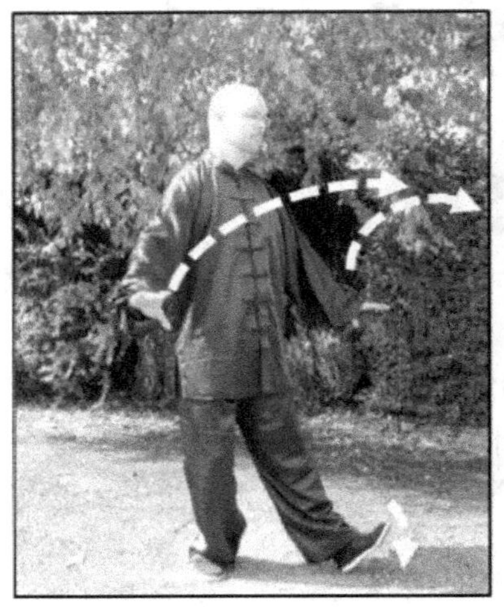 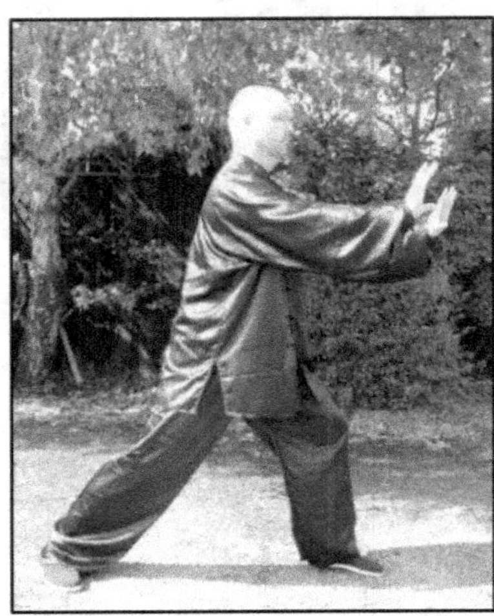

On completion, step back and repeat on the right side.

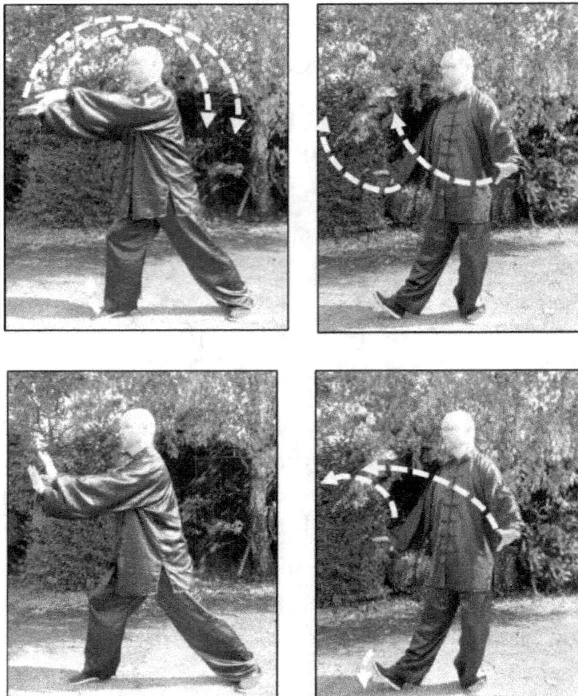

Posture 13. Flying Dove

On completion of the previous posture, step out on the left diagonal and as you push forward, sweep your palms forward then as you rock back, open them up. The hand movements are similar to Posture 2 but with a slightly more extensive and flowing action of the "flight" muscles. The footwork is the same as Posture 12.

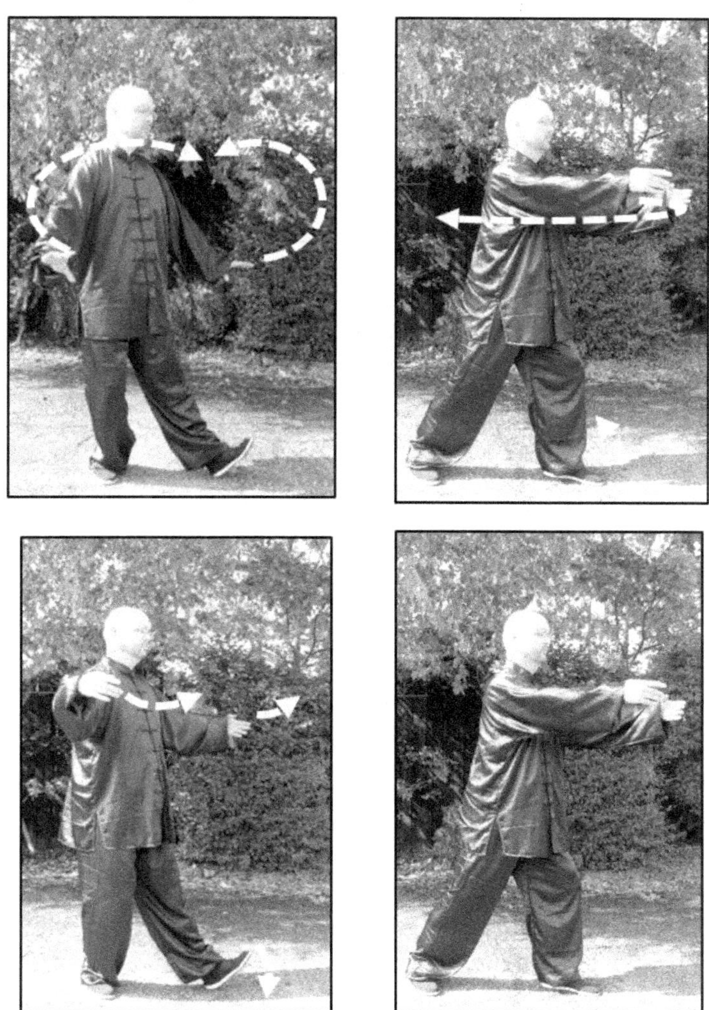

On completion, step back and repeat on the right side.

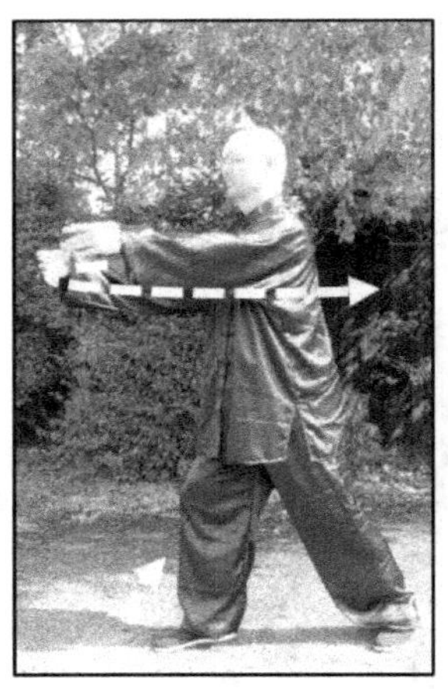 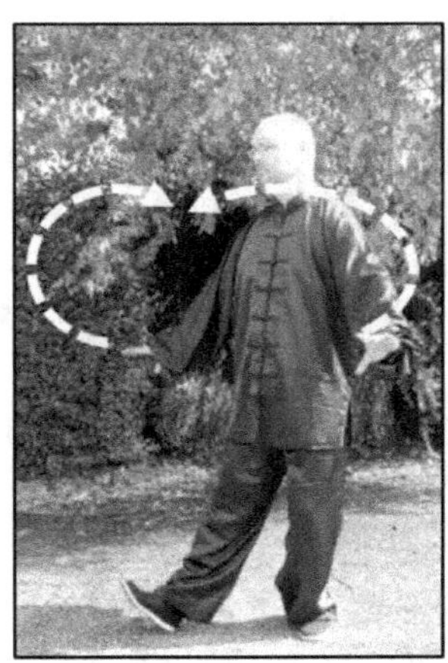

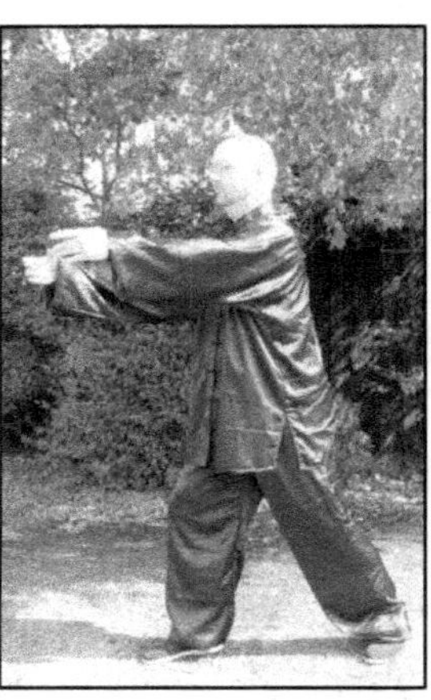 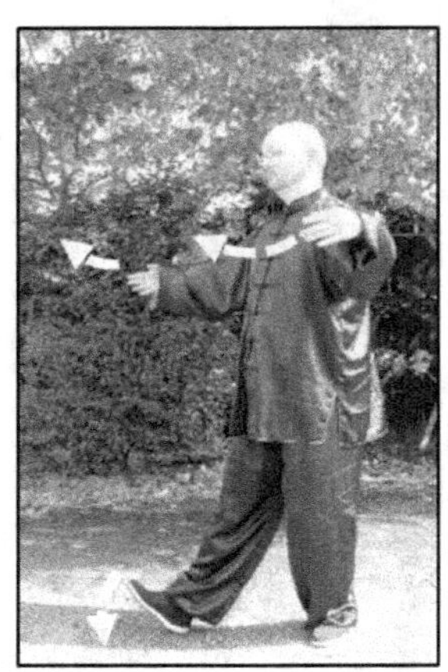

Posture 14. Charge with the Fist (punching)

The next posture is taken from basic martial arts training. It has a variety of benefits but an important function here is to be able to generate power from your root whilst maintaining stability. So, taking up the basic horse-riding posture, draw the relaxed fists back to the body at a comfortable level and then make a corkscrew punch forward with the left fist and draw it back to the hip. Alternate the slow punch left and right. Do this in slow and relaxed way but imagine you are punching with great power.

Take care not to tense the shoulders when punching (a common error when practising punching) and make sure you fully relax them between each punch.

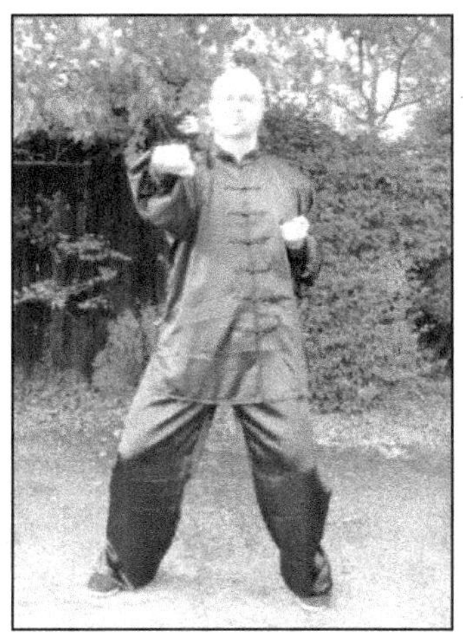 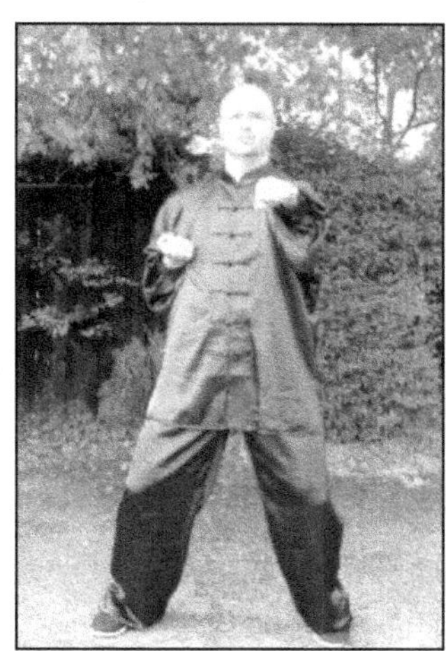

Optionally, if able and proficient, you might begin to widen and lower the posture, little by little. The picture below demonstrates the classic, lower *Hung Kuen* horse-riding posture. This is useful for developing strength, stamina, a strong root, proprioception, stability, and balance but should not be practised if you have a knee injury or if it causes pain.

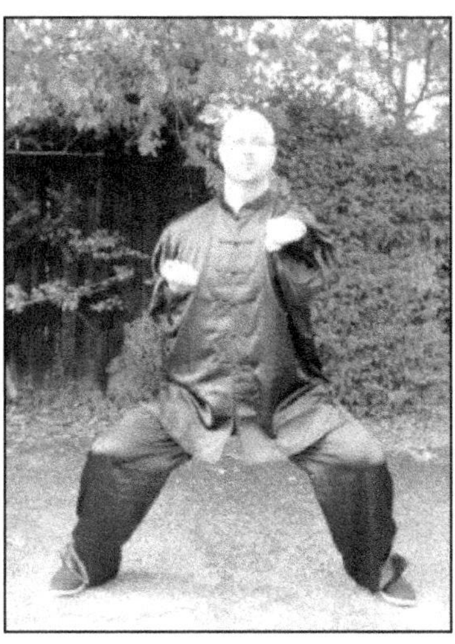

Posture 15. The Great Wild Goose Flying

In the normal or low horse-riding posture, sweep the arms down, across and up in a graceful arc, sinking as you sweep your "wings" down and raising when you sweep them up. You should visualise the graceful extension and power of a goose in flight.

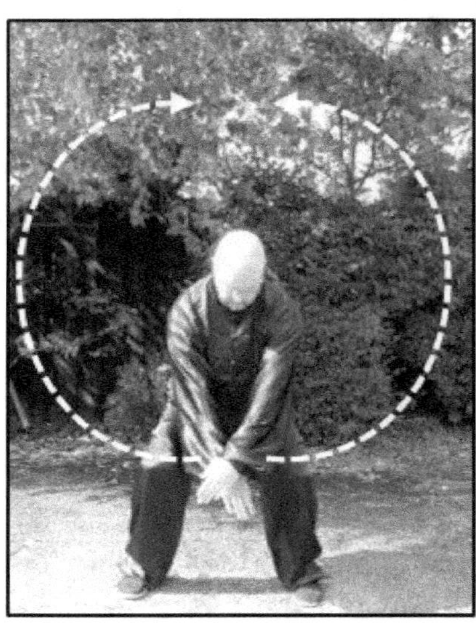 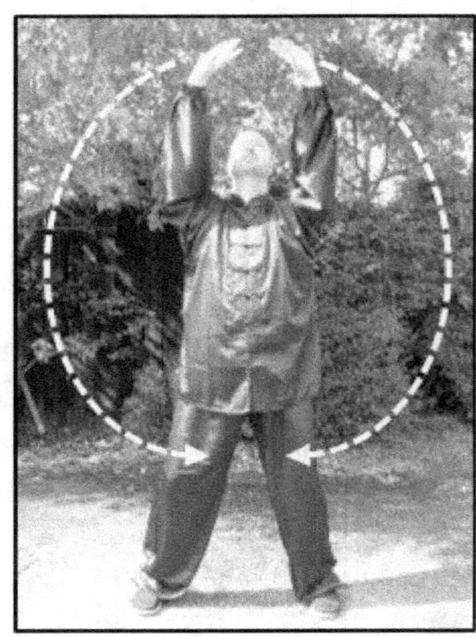

Posture 16. Rotating the Flywheel

From the final lowering of the previous posture, relax down and to the right (to make this comfortable, bend the knees as much as you wish) then continue relaxing as you sweep to the left and stretch up above your head or as high as you can. Continue circling in a clockwise direction as you relax down to the left.

Before rising, "put the brakes on" and reverse the movement circling in the anticlockwise direction using the stored momentum. Perform this movement slowly and carefully to avoid dizziness. When you develop a certain amount of flexibility you might wish to add a slight turn of the waist to the sideward/upward movement. Initially, to avoid strained ribs muscles, be careful not to overstretch upwards.

Be careful to do this slowly, stretching up but relaxing down. For the more experienced and able, the upward stretch can incorporate a careful extension of the spine.

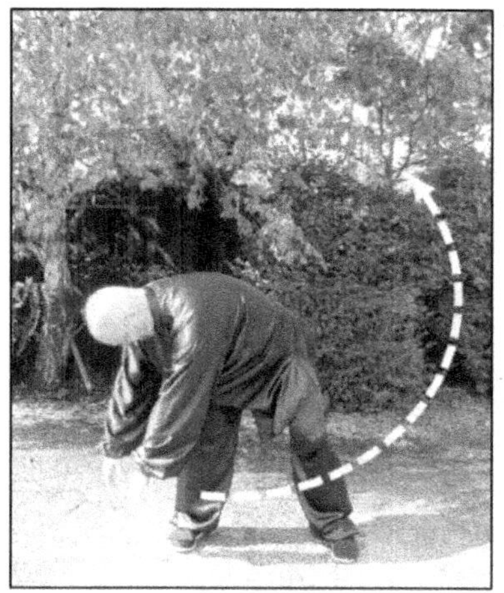 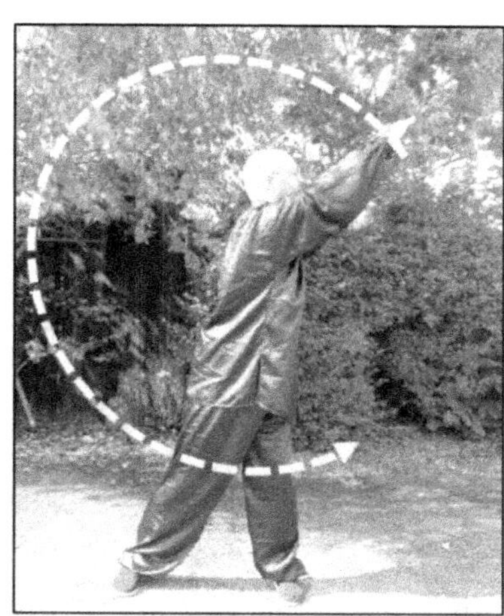

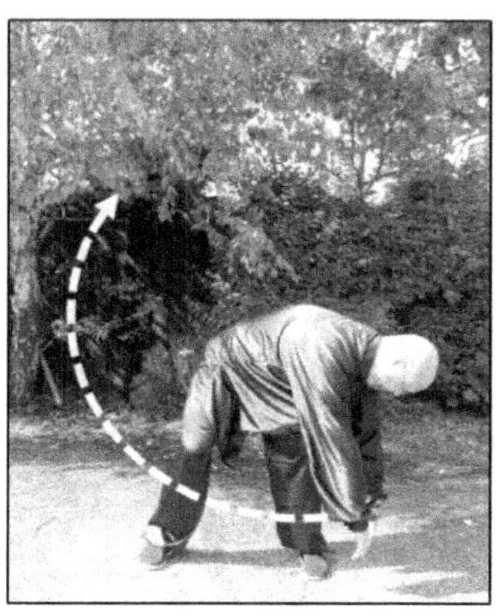 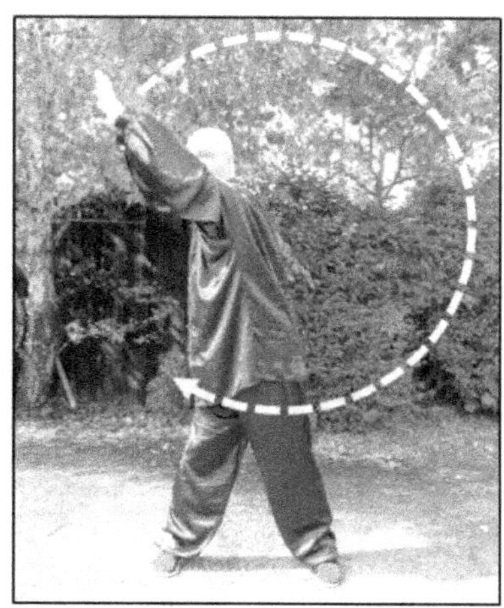

Posture 17. Bouncing the Ball While Marching

This exercise is effective for helping to maintain and develop balance and coordination along with reducing the common tendency toward valgus stress on the knee joint (and if you do it while waiting in a long bus queue, the queue in front will suddenly disappear!).

Raise and lower the left arm as in *Regulate the Breathing* posture but at the same time raise and lower the opposite knee, slowly and gracefully. Try to lower your foot gently, placing it back on the floor without any noise but correctly aligned. There are alternative ways to perform this posture, but I find this to be the best for coordination and balance training.

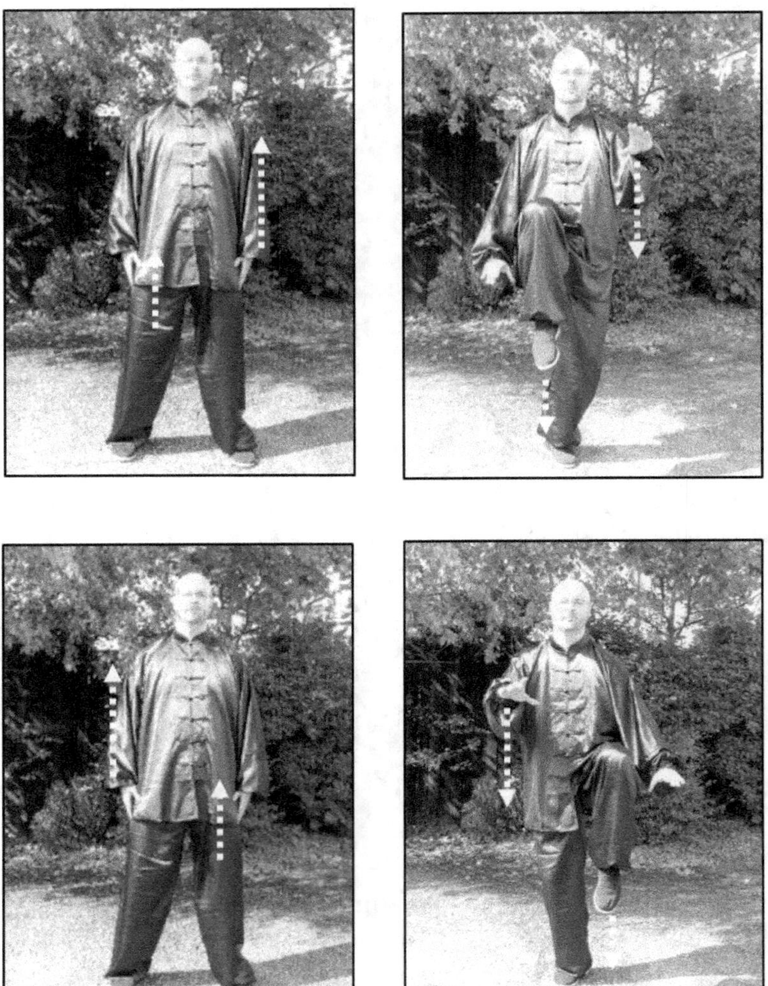

As there is a common tendency to raise the leg in a valgus (knock-kneed) manner with the foot everted (tilted outwards), try to ensure that you raise the knee up straight with the foot pointing slightly down and in line with the knee (as shown above).

Posture 18. Regulating the Chi

We began the form with *Regulating the Breath*. As we have now mobilised everything including our Chi, so things are hopefully flowing more actively and effectively, we now need to settle everything down so that the Chi and fluids are flowing and functioning optimally and will not become scattered and dissipated. To this end, we must now *Regulate the Chi*.

Whether or not you believe in Chi flow etc., this posture has general beneficial physical and mental effects. For example, it is useful for calming the mind and breath and fully relaxing the body after the exercises. In Western terms we might think of it as a warming-down exercise. In Chi Gung, there are particular visualisation techniques for this posture with regard to Chinese medical theory, but this requires instruction from an accomplished teacher. Here it is best to just pay attention to the breath. Using a cleansing breath as we did at the start of the form, breathe-in as you lift your hands (like you are using them to draw air into the lungs) and breath-out as you press the hands down (like you are pressing down on the abdomen, which in turn pushes the air out of the lungs). You are not doing a great deal, so take it slow and do not overdo the deep breath as it might cause dizziness. Repeat the same number of times as you repeated each posture, i.e., if you performed each individual posture 3 times, perform this 3 times also.

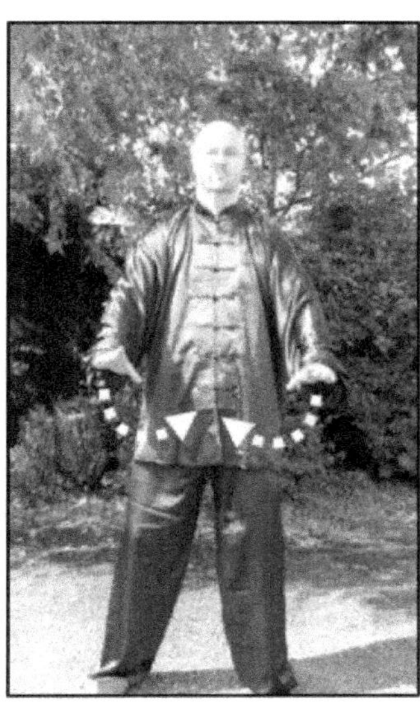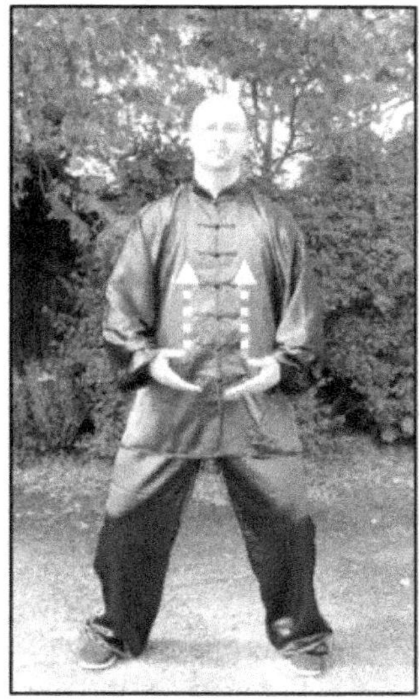

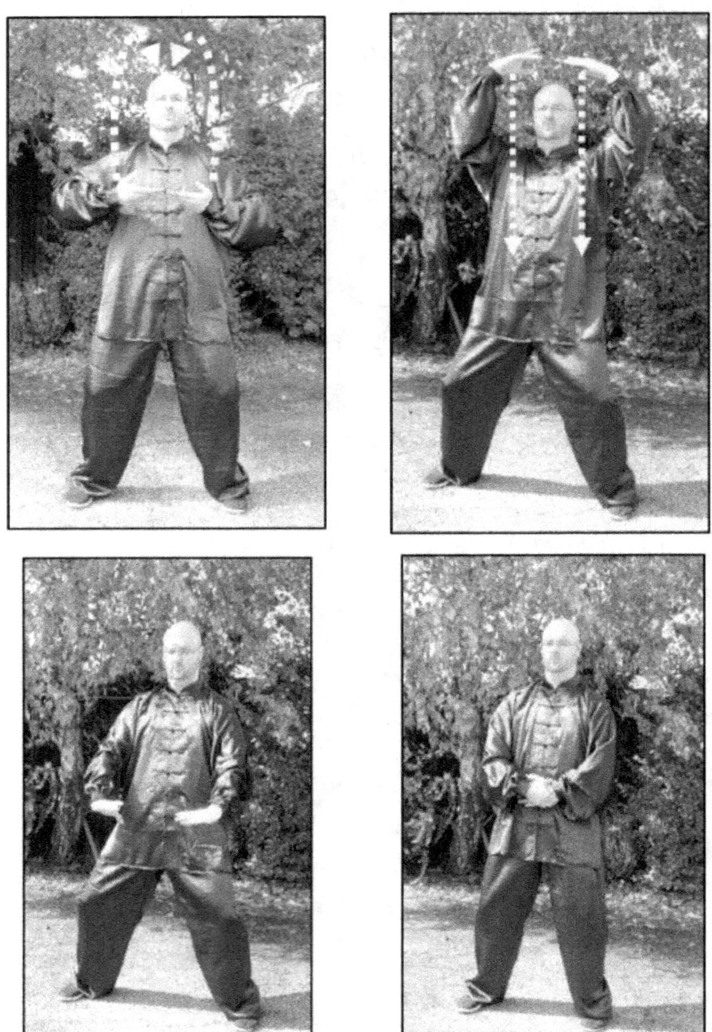

With the final in-breath, visualise the breath moving down to the *dantien* (just below the navel). At the same time, the hands are drawn in to rest at that point. Thus, you are closing in and settling everything down to your centre. Finally, let your breath calm to a natural relaxed state. Here you can either keep your attention at the *dantien* or on the calm breath moving in and out.

****

As with the previous set of mobilising exercises, these eighteen postures can be used as a stand-alone form. However, they are additionally effective if practised after the mobilising and stretching exercises. Furthermore, practising this form will also prepare you for practise of the slightly complex postures, transitions, and rhythmic nature of the more dynamic form of Chi Gung known as Tai Chi.

Although I have provided suitable instruction for the exercises to be relatively safe and beneficial, it is always best to obtain detailed instruction from a competent teacher when possible. Furthermore, the 18 postures can be appropriately adapted for seated persons with mobility issues. However, as with the standing postures, it is always best if a competent instructor is on hand to tailor the postures to meet the specific needs of the individual. This is perhaps more important for individuals with mobility issues.

18 Postures Tai Chi-Chi Gung – Seated

In the first edition of this book, I had decided for safety reasons not to present the following seated exercises because individuals with mobility issues have their own unique needs and therefore require individual assistance / instruction to adapt the postures appropriately. However, I realise that not everyone has access to a teacher and so, in this edition, I have presented an adapted version and provided some additional detail in the explanatory text. The postures are adapted from the latter standing form specifically to aid individuals who may not be able to stand for long periods. It is important to know your limitations and especially pay attention to the following important points.

Important Points for Seated Exercises.

- Seated exercise should be carried out in a secure chair that will not move or tip over when you are moving in any direction.

- Because you will be seated for this form, your root will be your feet and your backside so, other than for movements that require a slight upward lift, you should maintain a firm downward root from the feet and backside.

- For movements that require lowering the body forward, you should be especially careful not to exceed your limitations of strength, flexibility, and balance. If you are unable to lean forward, you could try to move forward slightly as much as you safely can. If you cannot do this, you should try simply to visualise moving forward. In addition, because you will be in a firm chair with no danger of tipping you can try to gently rock/push back into the chair.

- To incorporate movement and enhance the exercises, any stepping is carried out in a slow and somewhat exaggerated manner. As stepping while seated can be difficult and might, for some, cause a degree of strain on the low back, it is permissible to gain support by holding the arms or sides of the chair while stepping.

- Joint movements should be within physical and pain limitations. If for example you can only raise you right arm to the level of your chest without pain, then that is as far as you need to go, but then the left arm should be raised only to that same level. A key principle is relaxation in movement. Trying to move a painful joint beyond its limits (a technique for professionals) will only create tension. The theory for us is that by gentle repetition within our limitations, movement might be maintained and gradually improved.

NB Assuming you have already consulted your health care provider about the suitability of the exercises, if your immobility/disability entails loss of bodily control or balance, then it is advised that you avoid movement that could exacerbate your problem and cause injury, and certainly only perform them with the aid of an assistant/carer.

Posture 1. Regulating the Breath

Begin in a seated *Wu chi* posture (Review pages 4-7) with the correct spinal alignment as best you can. Then take some "cleansing breaths" so that you feel relaxed, comfortable, and rooted.

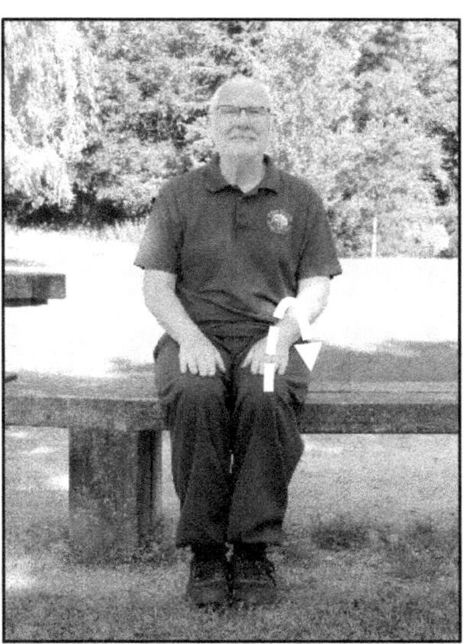

Now, lift the left leg up as high as you can (avoid pain or the need to rock or distort your spine and torso) with your toe pointing downwards, then move the leg out gracefully and slowly place the left foot on the floor in line with the right shoulder. In the same slow and graceful manner, step out with the right foot in line with the right shoulder. This is the basic seated horse-riding posture (*Mabu*). Rest your hands on you lap or arms of the chair.

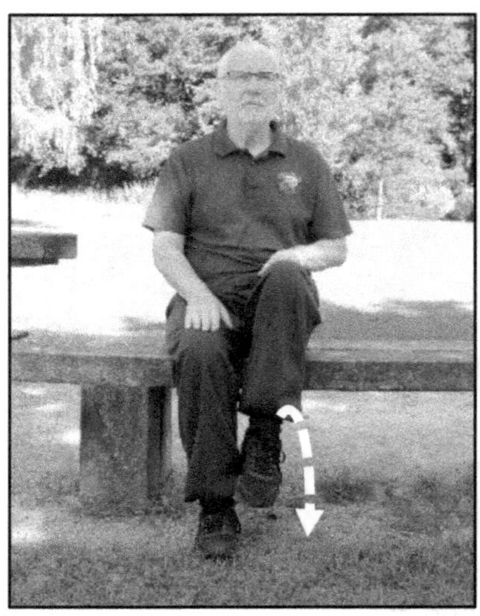 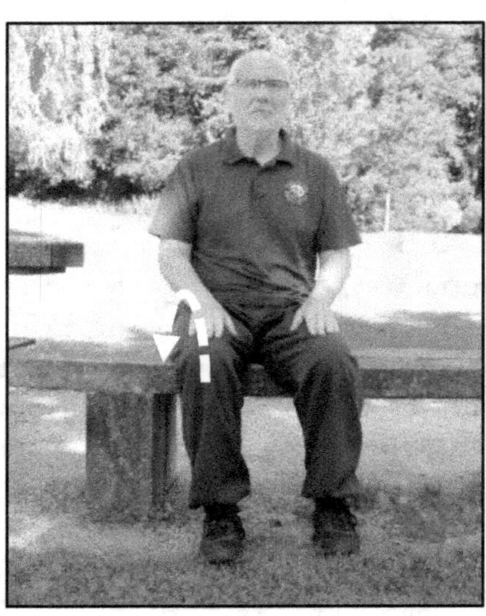

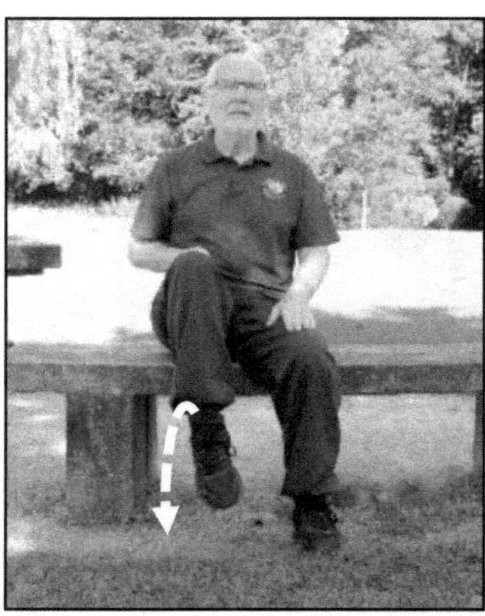 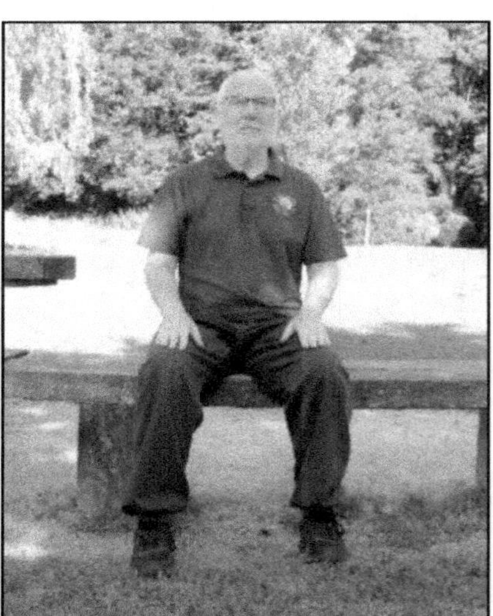

Next, breathe-in naturally as you raise the arms to shoulder height and breath-out as you lower them to the level of the *dantien*.

The hands describe an upward and forward arc then a downward, slightly inward arc. As you raise the arms, gently push down with your root. As you lower the arms, sink into the root, and relax.

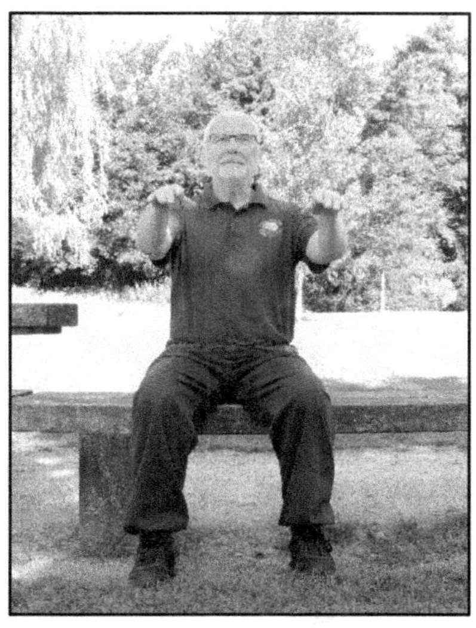 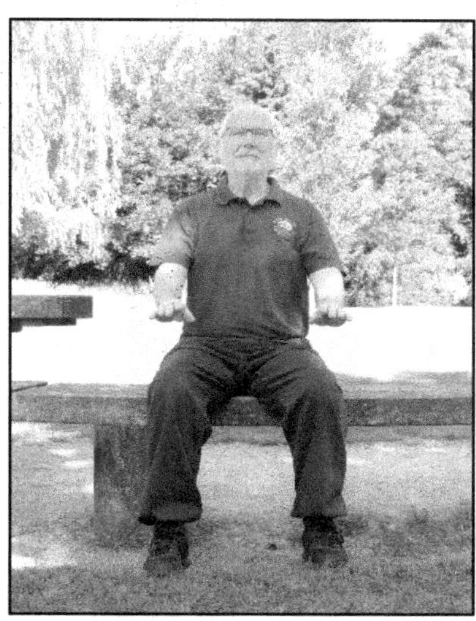

Posture 2. Opening the Chest

Flowing through from the previous posture, this movement has a similar quality and characteristic, but is more expansive.

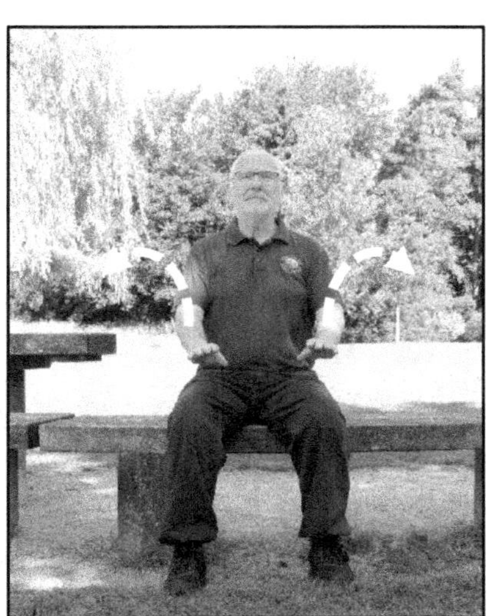 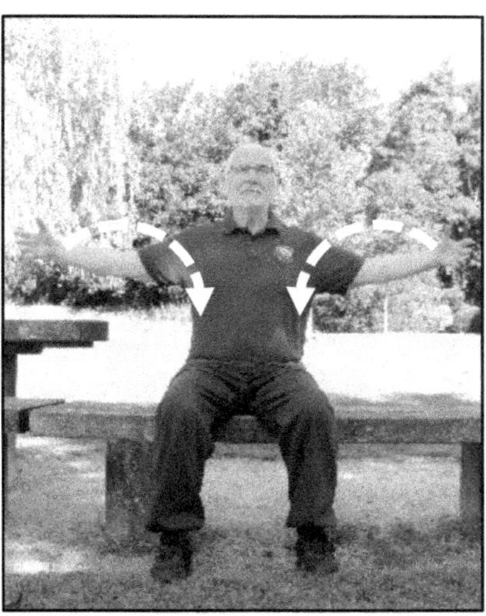

It is helpful to visualise a rising balloon pushing the palms up and expanding to push them apart. Then, you compress the balloon, pushing out the air to gently press it down to the resting position. As with the previous posture, when raising the arms, gently push down with your root then, as you lower the arms, sink into the root and relax.

Posture 3. Dancing with the Rainbow (left side)

Flowing through from the previous posture, visualise opening a rainbow above your head. Keep the shoulders relaxed as you relax into an upright but comfortable horse-riding posture.

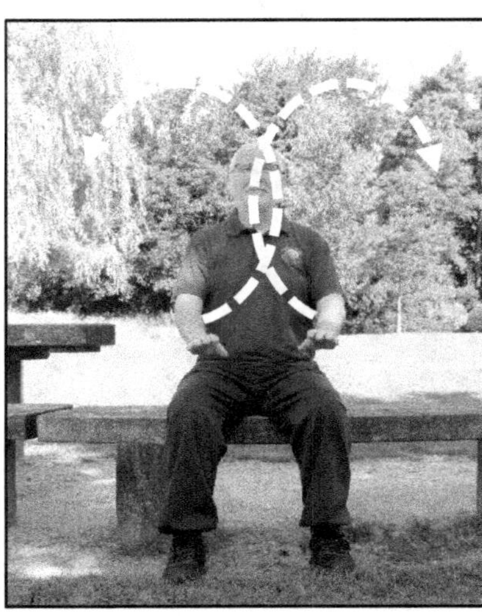 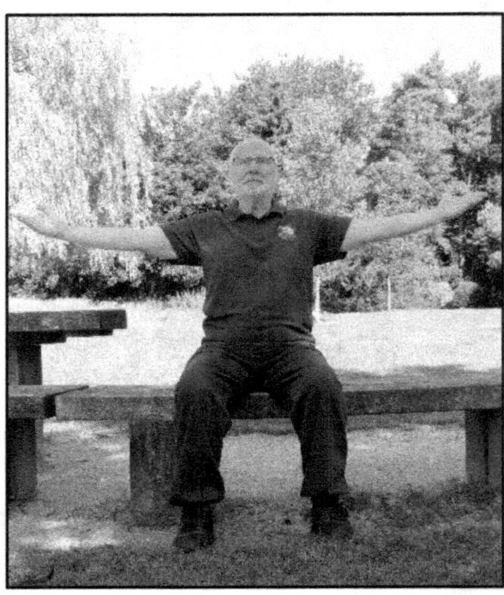

Now lift the left knee up as high as you comfortably can, without pain, with your toe pointing downwards. Move the leg slightly out and place down gracefully and slowly but this time with the foot pointing diagonally left.

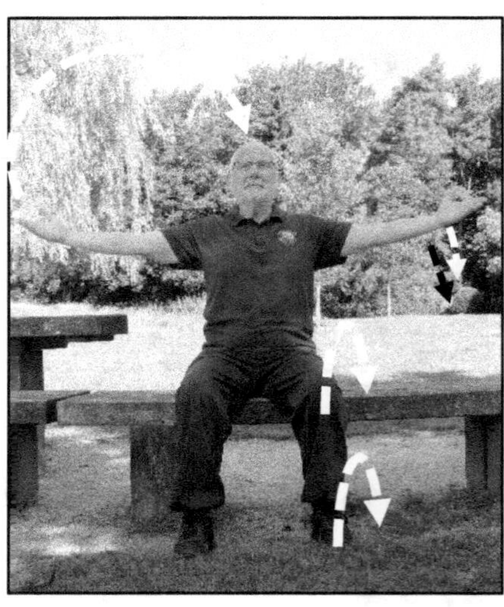 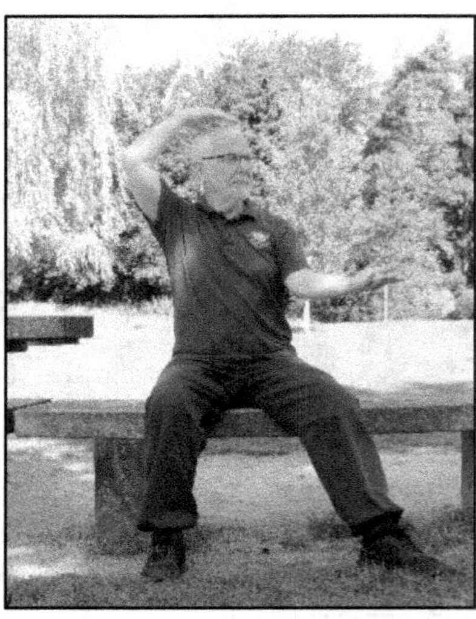

The outstretched foot only rests lightly on the floor while the rest of your body remains rooted on the chair this is the seated version of the *empty posture*. In coordination with the footwork, sweep the left hand out and down in an arc and the right hand just above the crown of the head or *baihui*. The arms and shoulders should be relaxed. Turn the head and body in the direction of the outstretched hand.

Dancing with the Rainbow (right side)

Following on from the left side posture: 1) step up, back, and in with the left foot, and then, 2) step up, out, and down diagonally with the right. With a flowing "Tai Chi" motion, complete the hand posture to the right side. The hands move as per the direction of the arrows in the diagrams. Repeat one or more times each side. Remember to keep the shoulders down and relaxed and remain rooted in the seat.

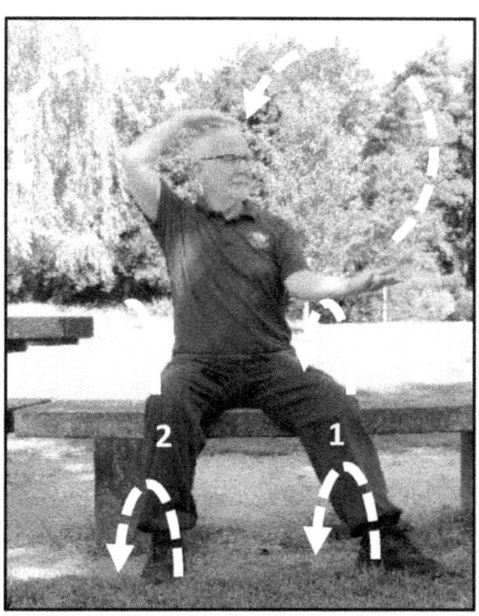
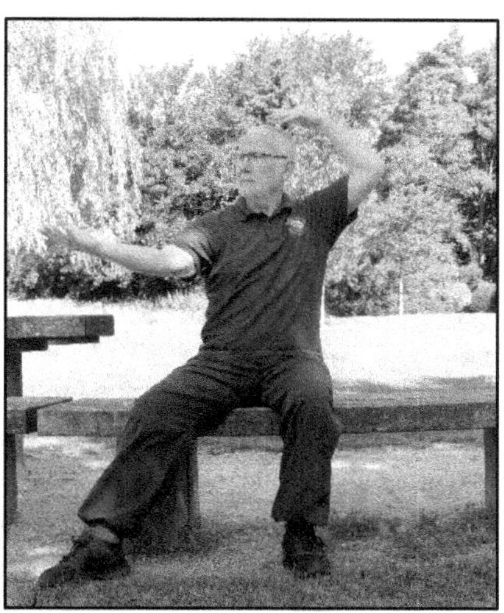

Importantly, as you raise the hand above the head, only raise it as high as you can so that it does not cause tension or pain and be sure to keep the shoulders relaxed. If possible, try to align the centre of the palm with the *baihui*.

When you have done sufficient repetitions (three on both sides is a useful number but once is ok if you are tired or are a beginner), bring your foot back to *Mabu* and sweep both hands out in a downward arc ready for the next posture.

Posture 4. Separating the Clouds

Continuing from the previous movement and maintaining the correct spinal posture, bend forward (Recall the important points above) as you cross the hands in front. Continue to sweep the arms across and upwards to cross above the head or as high as you can. Sweep them out in an arc and repeat. In Chi Gung, as a general rule, you should <u>stretch</u> upwards but <u>relax</u> downwards.

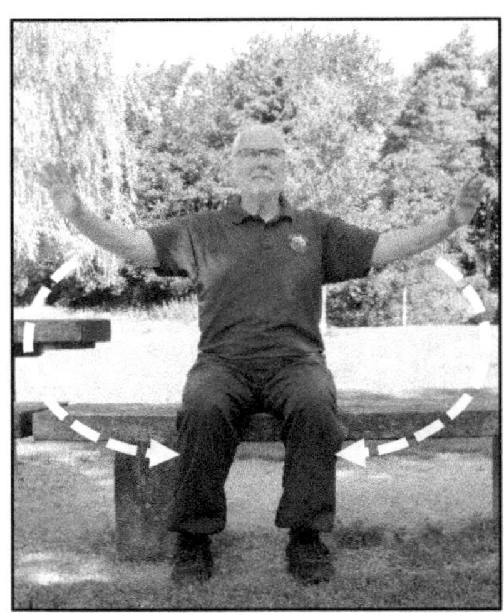

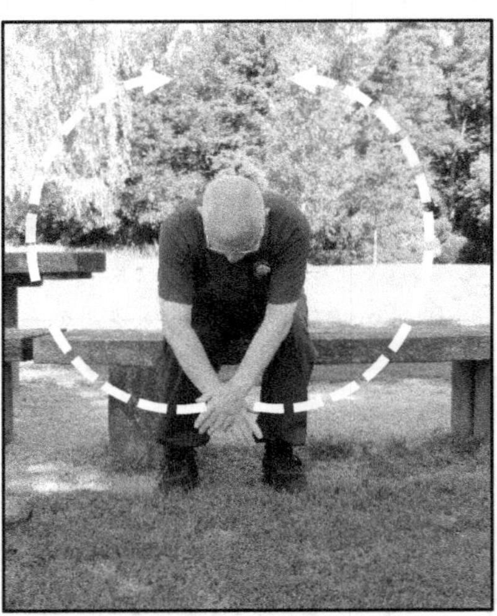

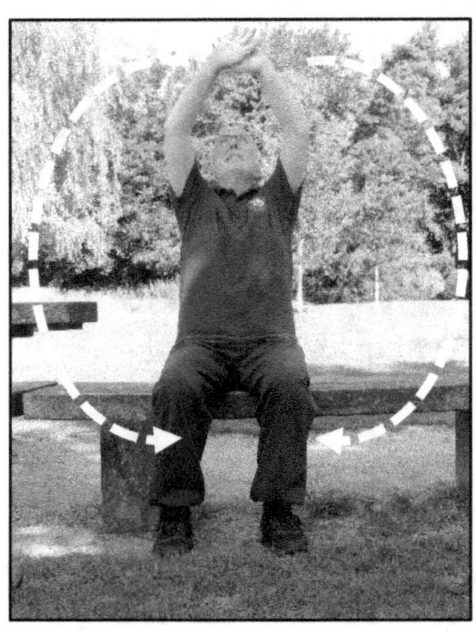

Posture 5. Reverse Reeling Arms (basic)

Although adapted from the moving posture of Tai Chi called *Step Backwards to Repulse the Monkey*, this movement is performed here in a strong seated horse-riding posture. The arms rotate in a smooth, flowing, and relaxed manner, a little like the freestyle swimming motion. In the basic movement you sweep the left arm out to the side, with the palm up, then gentle push forwards to the centre finally "settling the wrist", which means tilting the heel of the palm forwards emulating a martial palm strike.

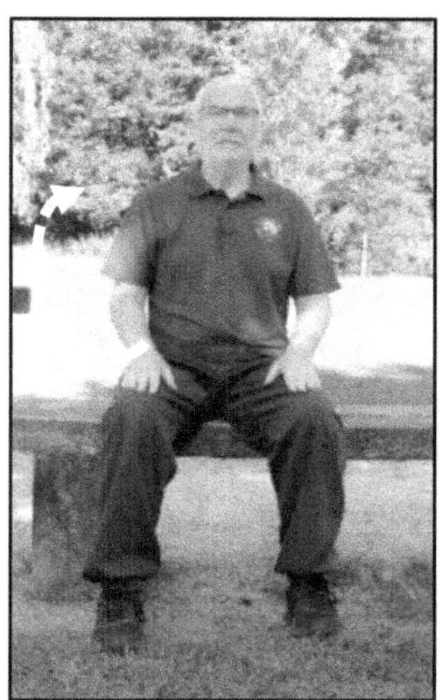 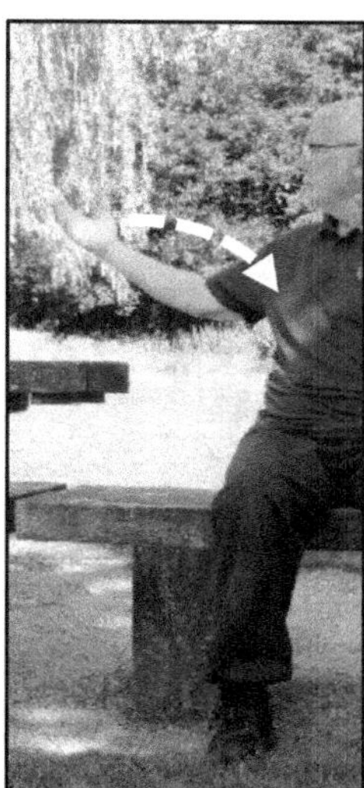 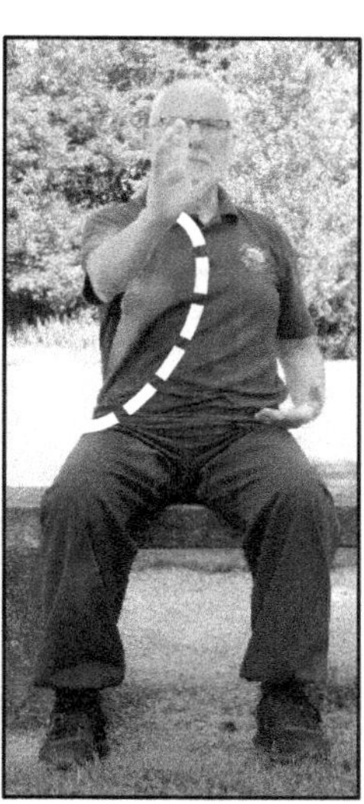

Repeat the desired number of times and then repeat on the opposite side. When familiar, alternate: left then right, etc. When you can perform this easily with a relaxed shoulder movement, incorporate turning of the waist and head as shown in the mid diagram above.

Reverse Reeling Arms (advanced)

If you wish, when familiar with the basic movement, from the basic posture, lift both hands with the palms upward, as shown in the photo below - the left hand to the front and the right hand to the side, then pull down the left hand along your centreline as you push the right forward "settling the wrist". Avoid undue raising of the shoulders and elbows. Repeat on both sides.

Once familiar with the movement you can coordinate a loose and relaxed waist movement as shown below.

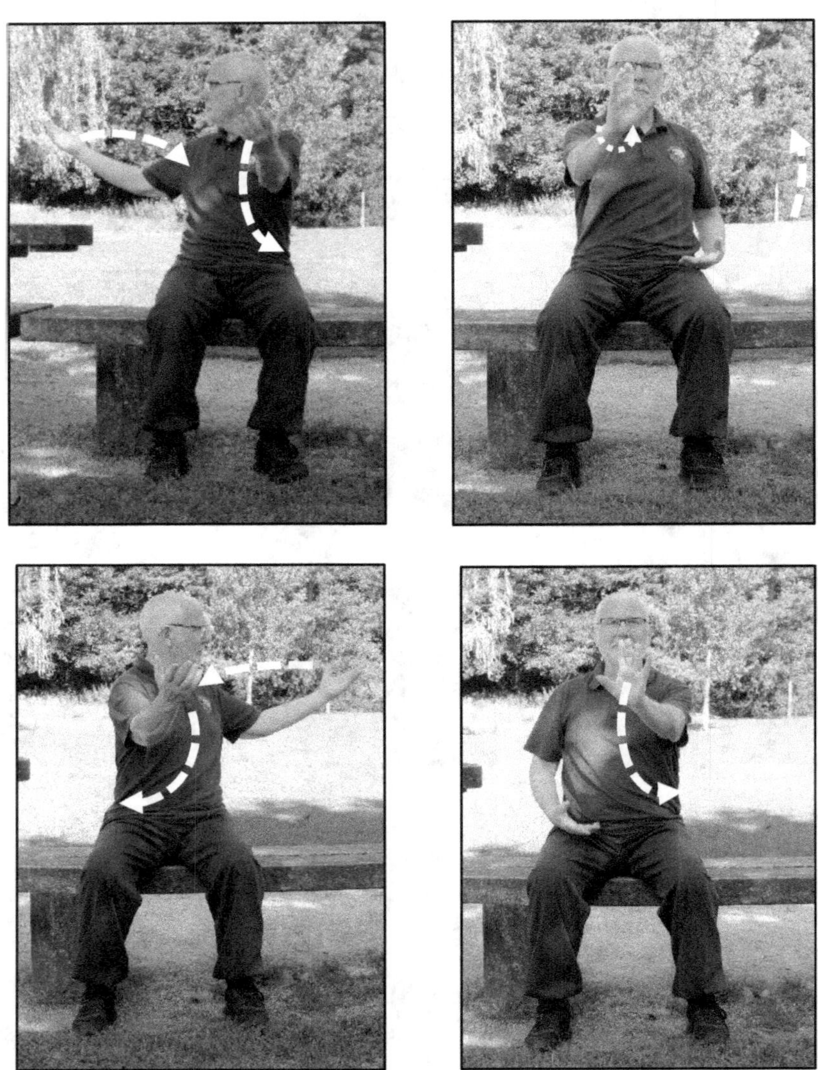

Posture 6. Rowing the Boat in the Centre of the Lake

Continuing from the previous posture, perform a rowing-like movement by sweeping both arms in an arc - outward, backward, and upward to then make a light fist at the shoulders. Then, relax forward and push the fists forward and down (like rowing a boat). Once again sweep the arms back up as you rise ready to repeat the movement and as the hands move backwards open the fists into the Tai Chi palm. Press down the palms to finish. For this seated exercise it can be useful, on raising back up to seated position, to apply some backward pressure on the chair (provided it is performed in a secure chair).

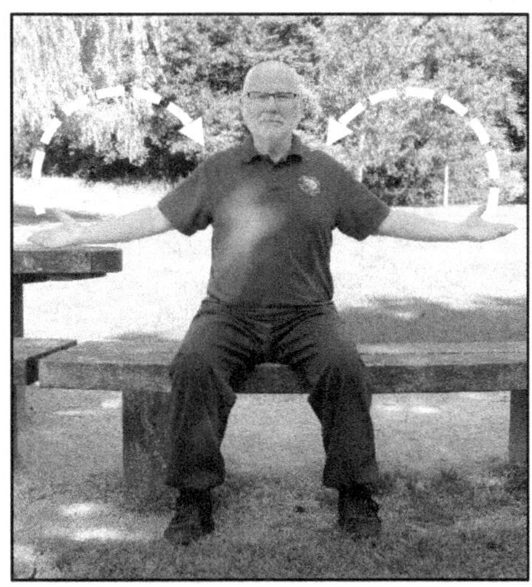

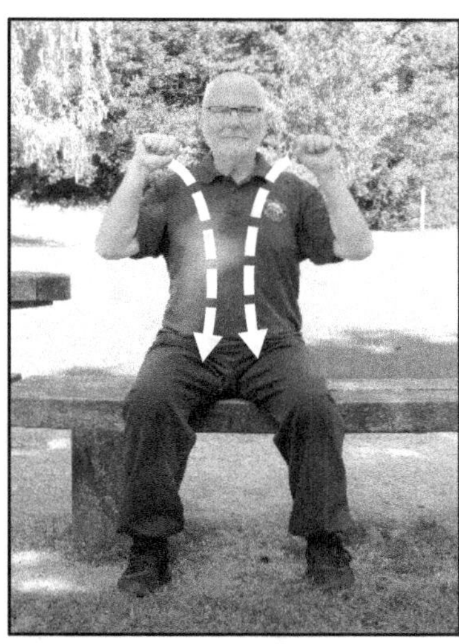

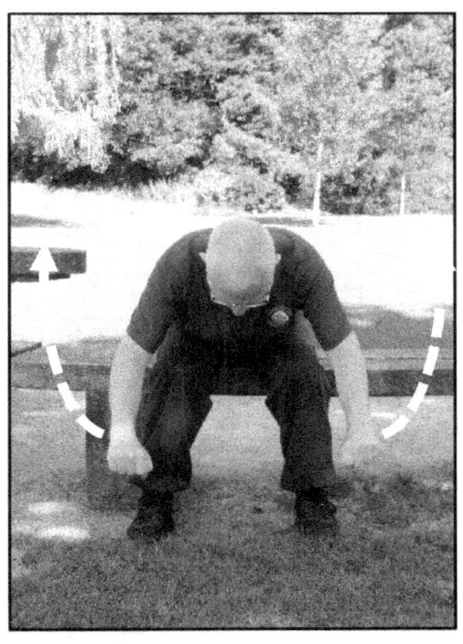

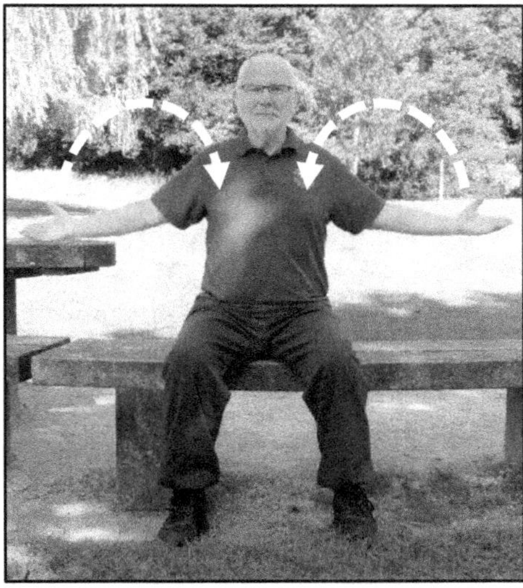

Posture 7. Supporting the Ball in Front of the Chest/Shoulder

Continuing from the previous posture, visualise catching a ball in front of the *dantien* and raising it across the body, left then right.

As you raise the right-hand palm-up to the left side, at the same time, raise the right heel keeping the ball of the foot on the floor. You gently turn your body as you stretch to the side but then relax when sinking back into the horse-riding posture and lowering the raised heel. Keep the waist loose and relaxed. Repeat an equal number of times left and right.

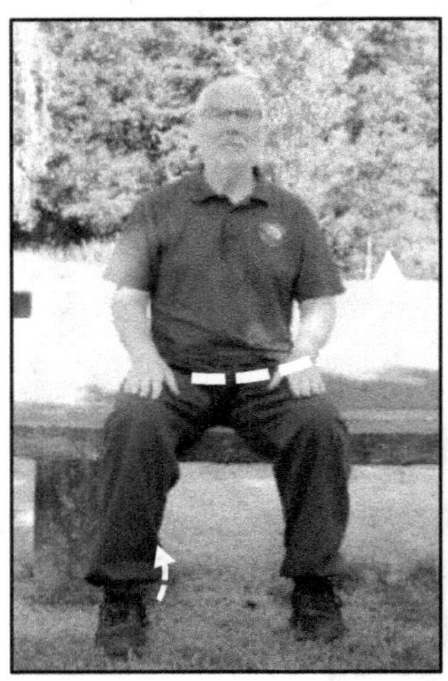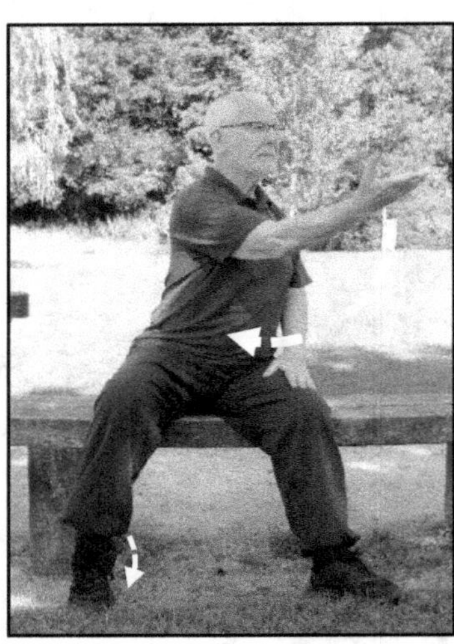

As with most of the movements this should be performed slowly and gracefully with a gentle side-to-side rocking motion.

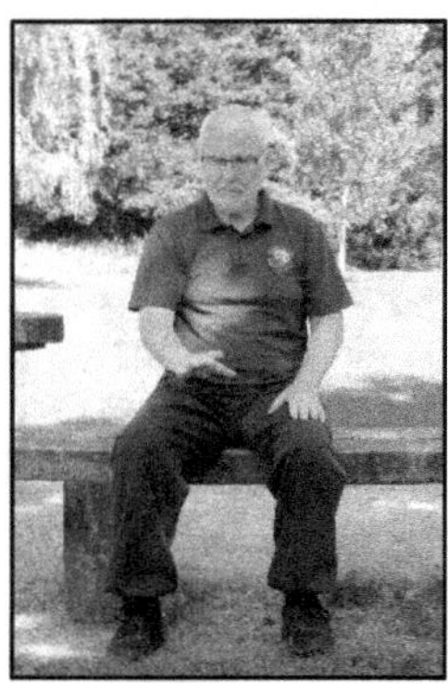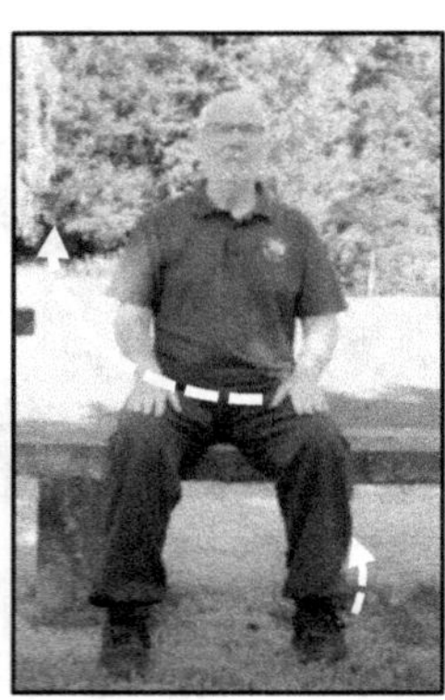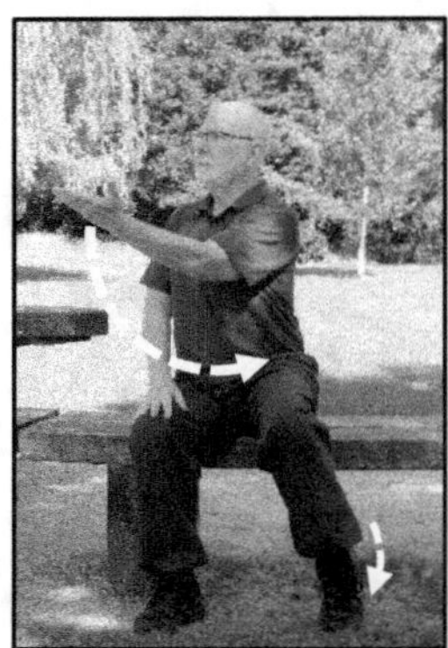

Posture 8. Turn the Body to Gaze at the Moon

Continue from the previous posture performing it in a similar vein, one side then the other, but now visualise holding the ball in both hands and raising it across the body and up. If capable, turn to gaze up between the hands. Take care not to overstretch at first as this might strain the rib muscles. When you become more flexible you can begin to turn slightly to the rear. If able, as you raise the arms, lift the heel on the opposite side keeping the toe and ball of the foot firmly rooted. Then relax when sinking back into *Mabu* as you lower the raised heel.

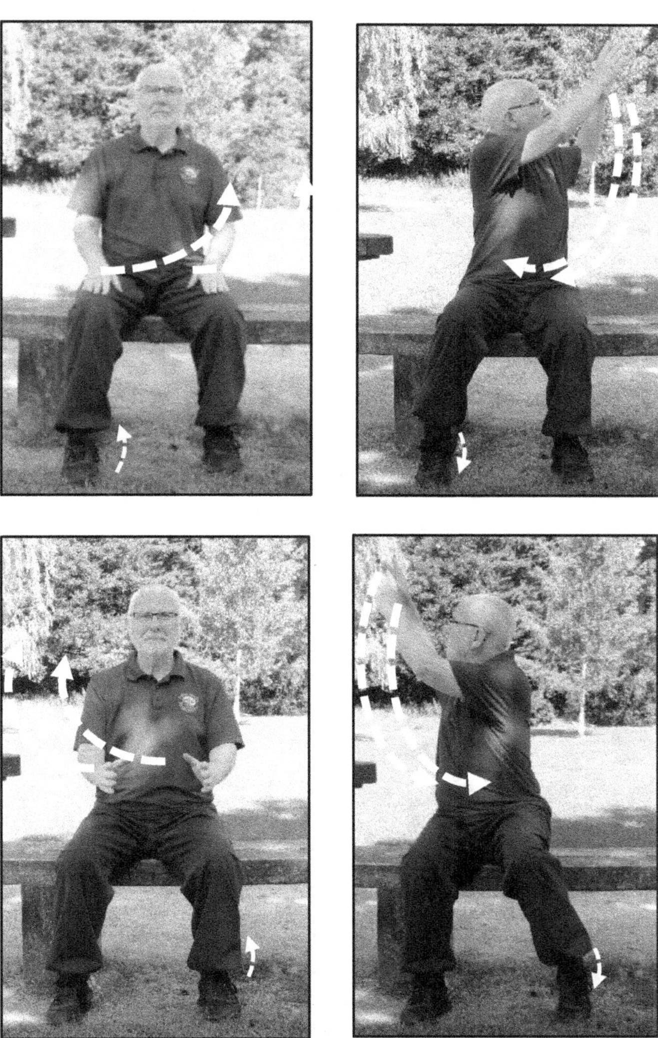

Posture 9. Turning Waist and Pushing Palm

Sitting in the horse-riding posture, draw the hands in to make a fist just above the hips. Establish the feeling of a strong root in the backside and feet. Open the left fist into a splayed palm and push forward and slightly upwards. Without allowing the palm to drift, turn your body to the right and then turn the head further to look behind (within your limitations). Now, relax and pull the left hand back to make a fist just above the hip then push the right palm forward and turn the body and head to the left. Again, your body will try to find the easiest way to do this by twisting the thigh and flexing the lumbar spine in a contorted manner, avoid this as much as possible.

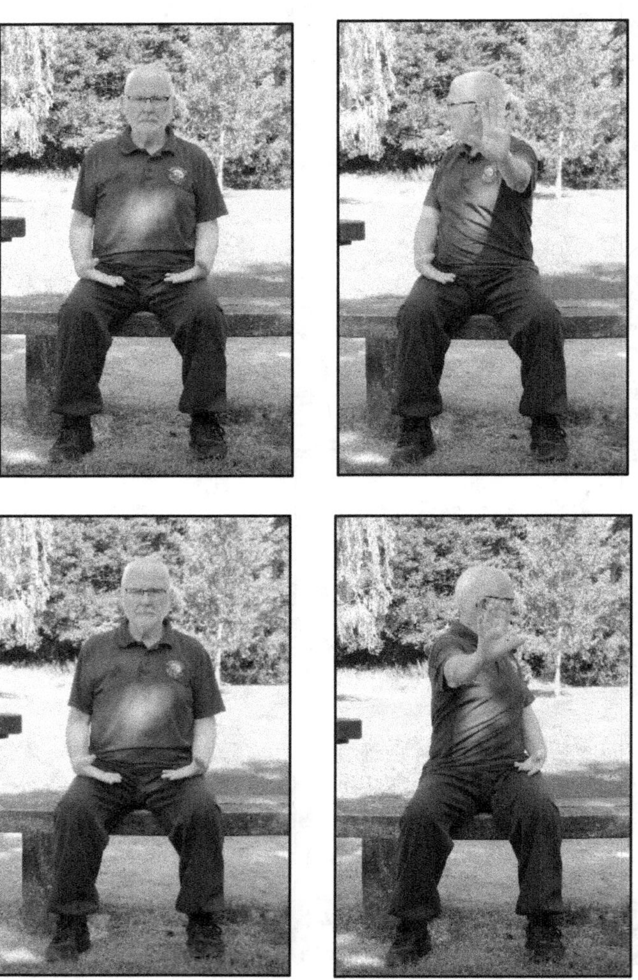

Posture 10. Hands Drifting in the Clouds

Initially, it might be helpful to practise this posture one side at a time. Following on from the previous posture, swirl the left palm anti-clockwise across the front-lower-body and upwards, then continue swirling the palm backwards across the front-upper-body. The shoulder girdle, wrist and elbow should remain relaxed. Repeat.

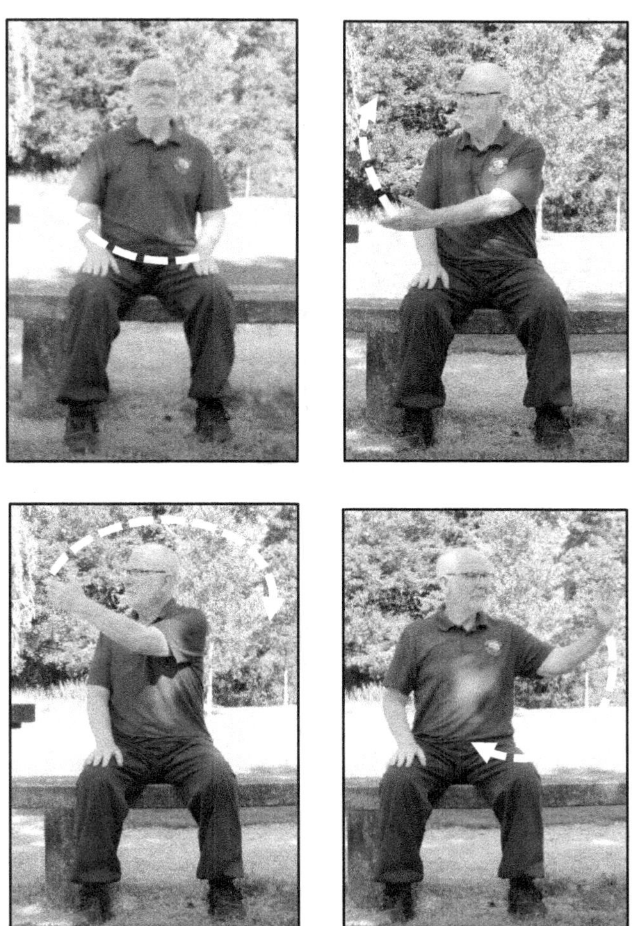

Now perform the movement clockwise with the right hand. As the hands brush down and in, the wrist extends, as the hand sweeps up and outward, the wrist flexes. You should also try to incorporate a relaxed waist movement from side to side. Try to visualise a lightness of the movement as though you are swirling cloud formations.

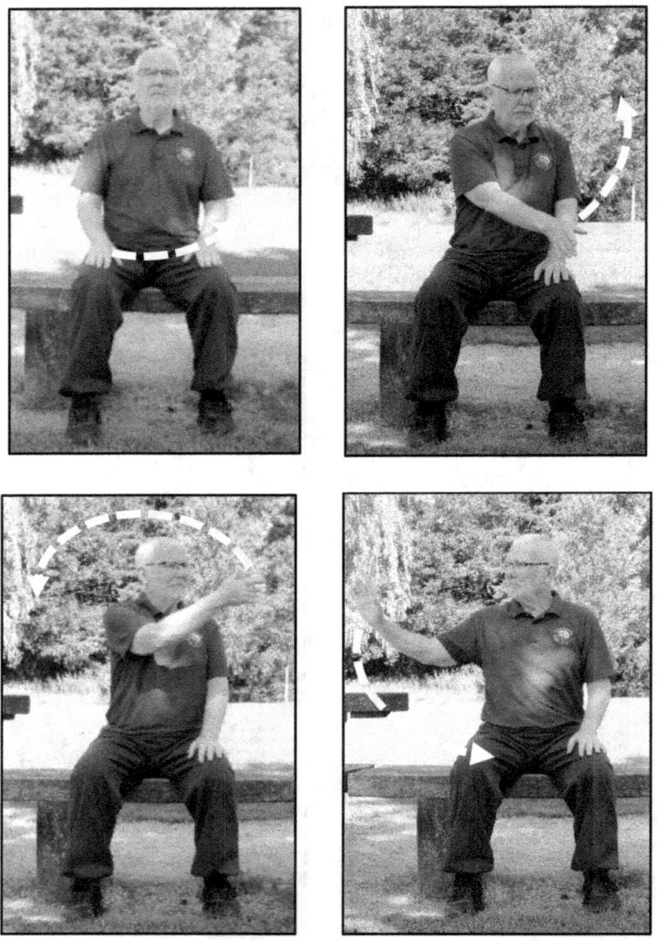

Once you are used to the movement, coordinate the hand movements on both sides as shown below. The left hand moves anti-clockwise, the right hand moves clockwise.

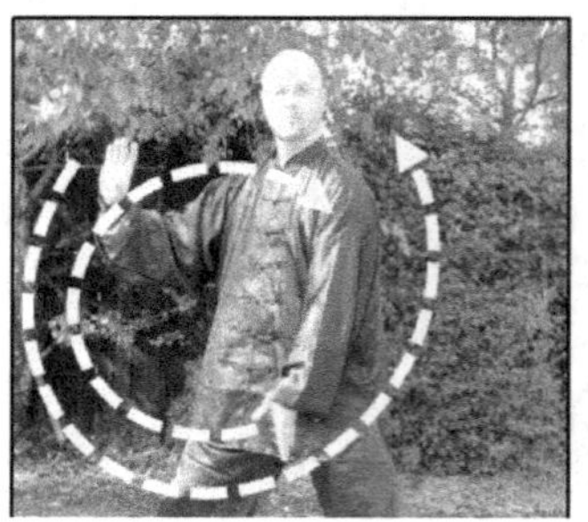

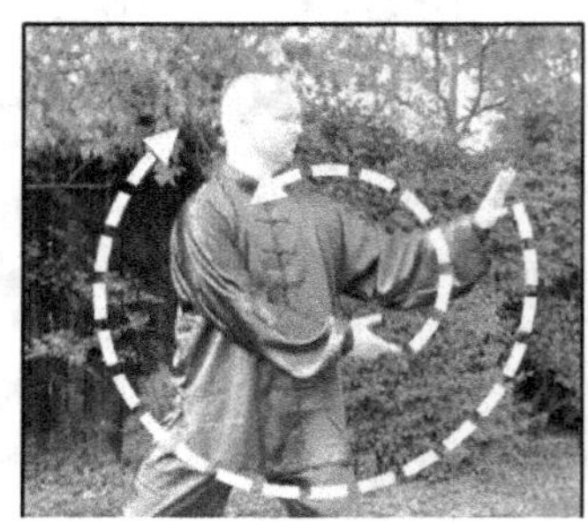

Posture 11. Dredging the Sea and Looking at the Sky

Following on from the previous posture, purposefully, but slowly and gently, step to the left, slightly on the diagonal. Then, remaining firmly seated, carry out hand movements similar to those of posture 3 - *Separating the Clouds* but more extensive and in the direction of the left foot. As you shift forward (within your limitations), relax the spine as much as possible. In addition to the general function of these exercises, this posture enables comfortable stretching and relaxation of the vertebral muscles and joints. This being the case, you should, at first, avoid excessive bending until the muscles develop some degree of strength and flexibility.

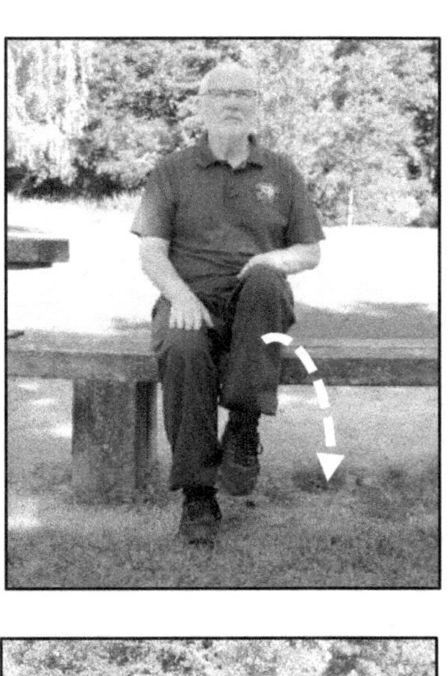
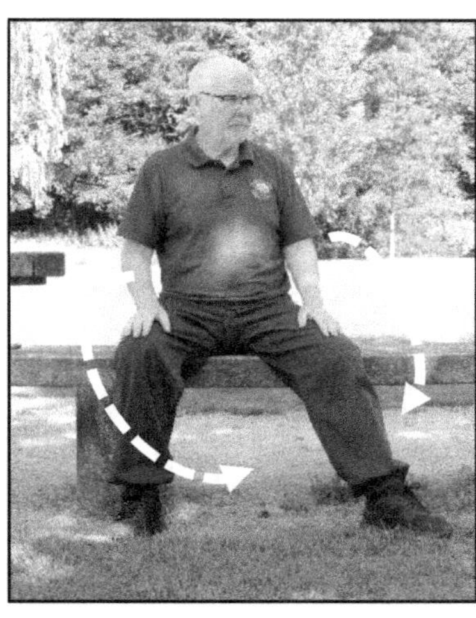
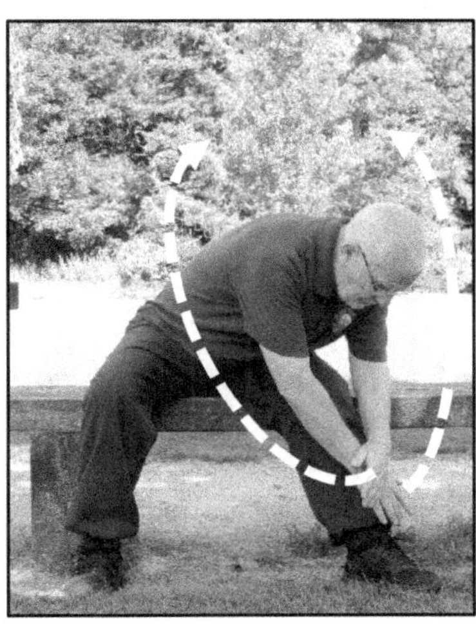
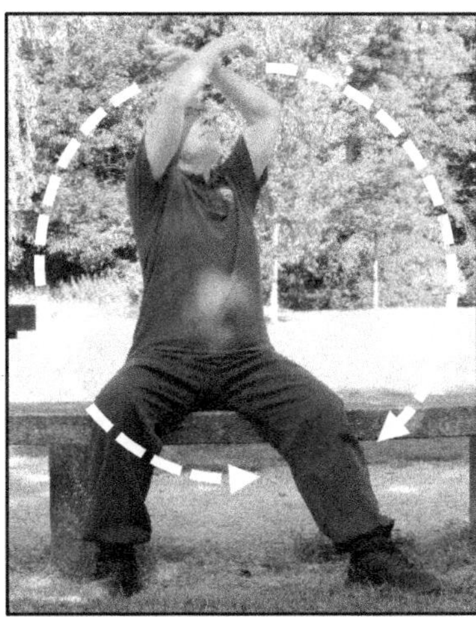

As you rise, support the lumbar spine by first shifting your weight to the backside. Try to avoid lunging upwards, curl the spine upwards by rooting in your seat and pushing up from it. This will avoid an unhealthy shearing movement of the lumber area. To complete the movement, stretch the arms crossed upwards then spread them outwards. As you reach down imagine you are looking deep into the sea and dredging the seabed. As you raise up imagine your hand are reaching up to the sky and separating clouds

On completion, step back and repeat on the right side as shown below.

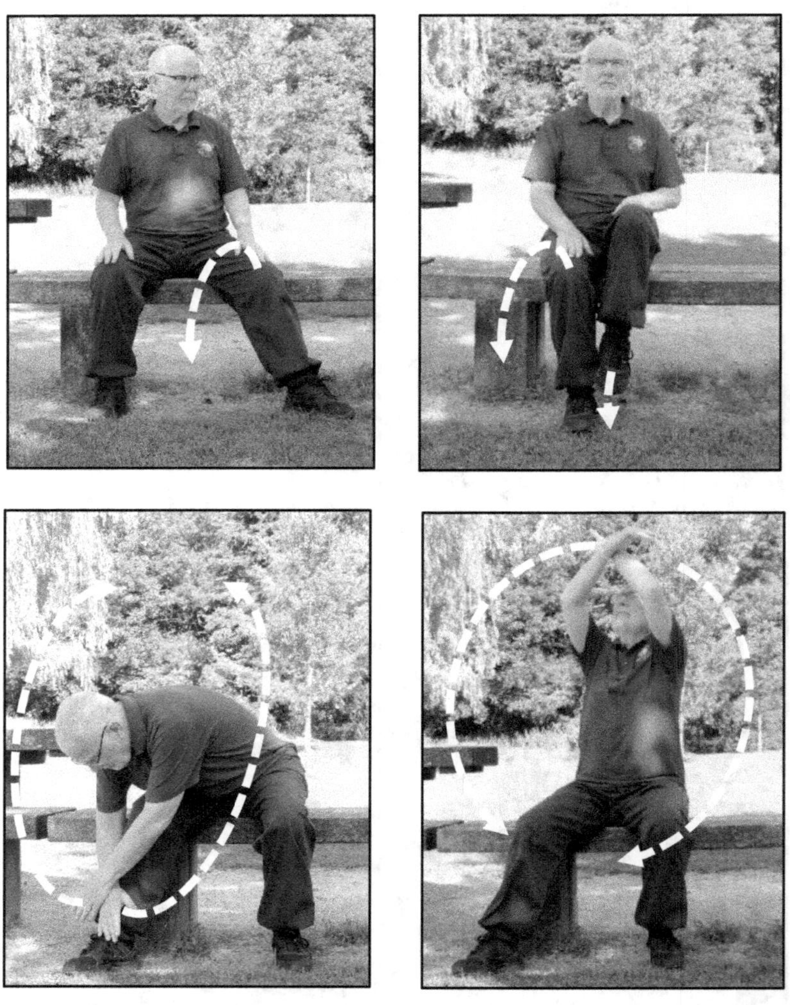

Posture 12. Pushing the Waves

Remember that at any point in the whole form, it is fine to rest between postures but if you are able, each posture should flow into the next. In this posture you must use a little more visualisation. As with the previous posture, step out on the left diagonal but now sweep your arms up as though you were catching the crest of a big wave coming toward you. Go with the flow of the wave by riding it back and then when its energy is guided down into your root, use this stored energy to push the water back out to sea.

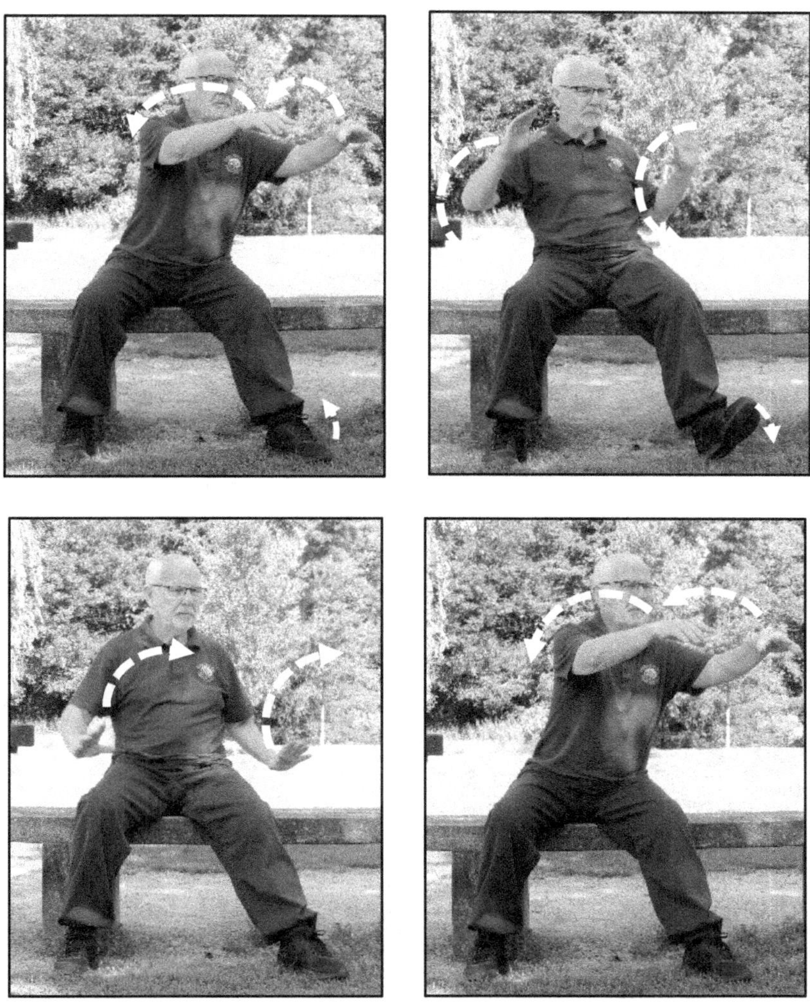

As you rock backwards lift the toes of the outstretched foot and stretch the left leg. Place the toes down again before you push the wave. As always, the rocking and pushing should be smooth, flowing, and relaxed. Remember to ensure the chair you are using is solid and stable.

On completion, as in the stepping action of Posture 11, step back with the left foot and step out with the right and repeat Pushing the Waves, this time on the right side.

Posture 13. Flying Dove
On completion of the previous posture, step back to the basic posture then step out on the left diagonal and as you push forward, sweep your palms forward then, as you rock back, open them up. The hand movements are like Posture 2 but with a slightly more extensive and flowing action of the "flight" muscles. As you flow backwards and forwards, the raising and lowering of the lead foot is the same as Posture 12.

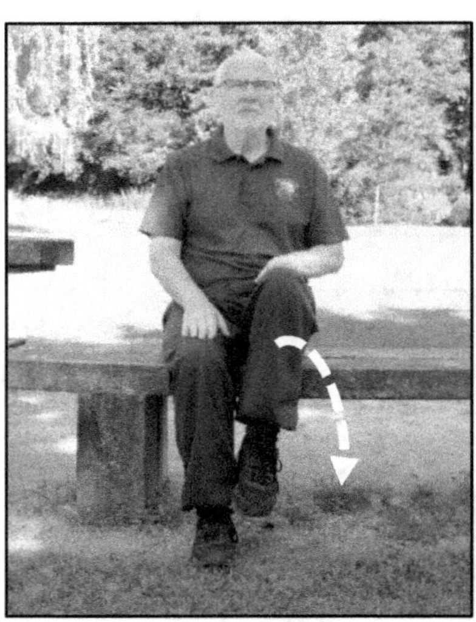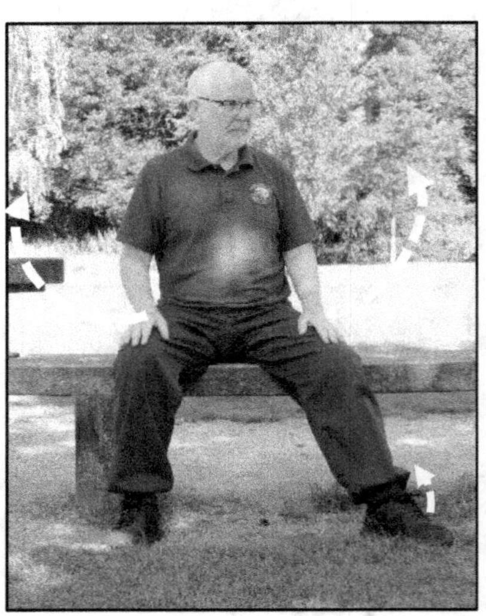

As you rock forward and backward the movement of the arms are coordinated and flowing. The motion is like the action a of dove in flight so you will be using your "flight" muscles somewhat, ensuring you engage and disengage the shoulder blades, opening and closing the chest, condensing, and expanding. The fingers are positioned in the "Tai Chi palm" and emulate open flight feathers.

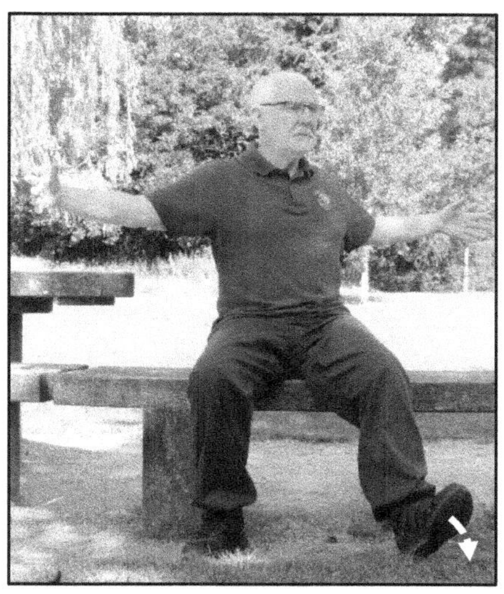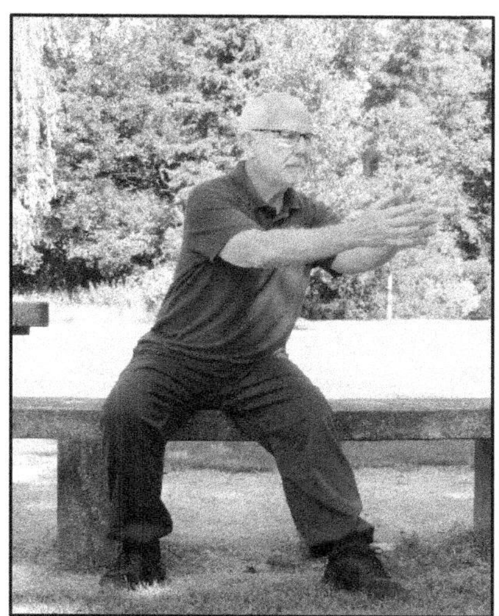

Step back and repeat the actions on the right side.

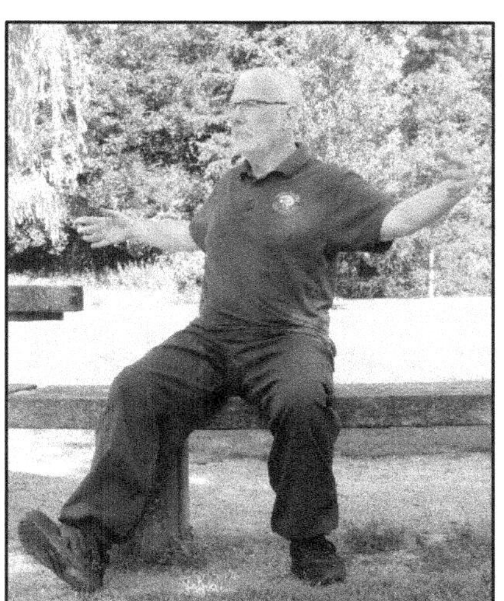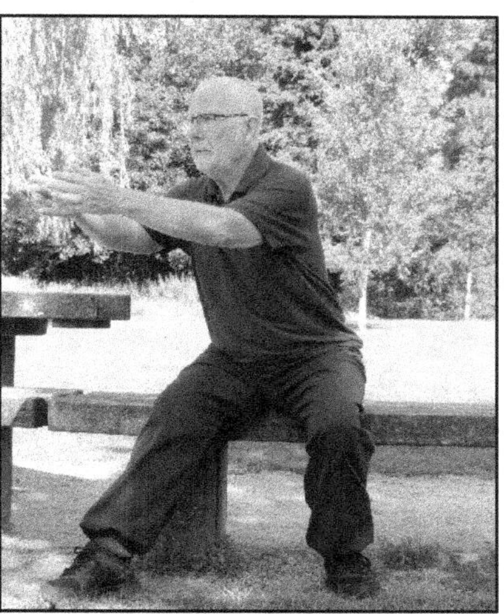

Safety Reminder: When performing these and other actions, ensure you are in a secure chair. If you feel unstable, or dizzy when performing these actions, you should cease until such a time as you are able to do them safely or until you have appropriate assistance or personal advice.

Posture 14. Charge with the Fist (punching)

The next posture is taken from basic martial arts training. It has a variety of benefits and is an amphoteric movement to balance the yin/yang energies but an important function here is to be able to generate the feeling of power from your root whilst maintaining stability. This feeling should be maintained as your fist "charges" forward.

So, from the previous movement, step back to the basic seated horse-riding posture, draw the relaxed fists back to the body at a comfortable level. In the standing form the root is in the feet but here you should feel a strong foundation in the feet and backside. Usually, the level of the resting fists depends on the martial style but here it is appropriate to hold them at the level shown in the photo. This is basically training in striking with the fist so make a corkscrew punch forward with the left fist and then draw it back to the hip. Then do the same with the right fist. Alternate the slow punch left and right. Do this in a relaxed way but imagine you are punching with great power. Take care not to tense the shoulders when punching (a common error when practising punching) and make sure you keep them level and fully relax them between each punch.

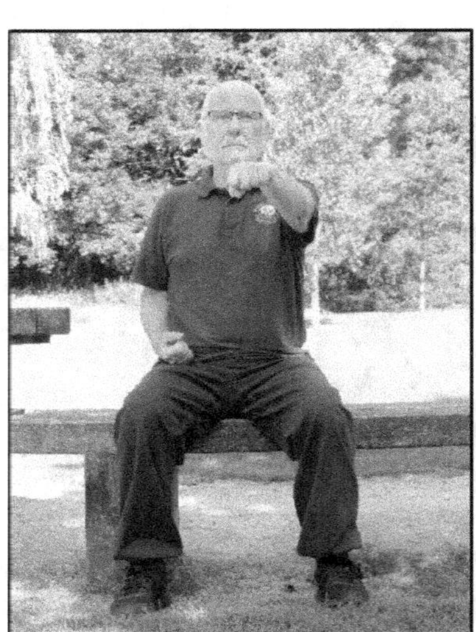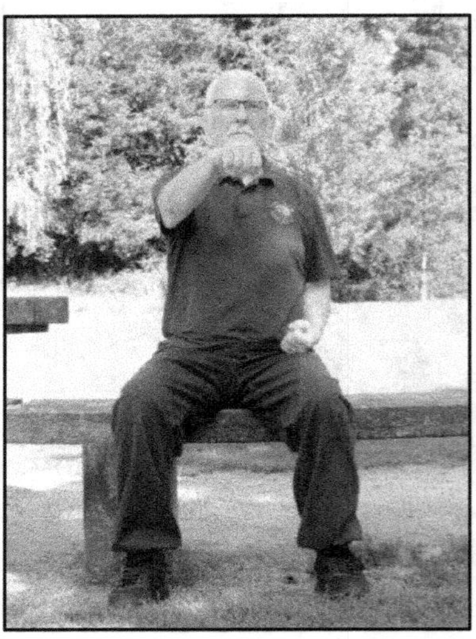

Although the movements are performed slowly and smoothly one should try to develop a feeling of confidence, strength, and stability.

Posture 15. The Great Wild Goose Flying

From the previous movement, return to the seated horse-riding posture, sweep the arms down, across and up in a graceful arc, sinking as you sweep your "wings" down and raising when you sweep them up. You should visualise the graceful wing extension and power and grace of a wild goose in flight.

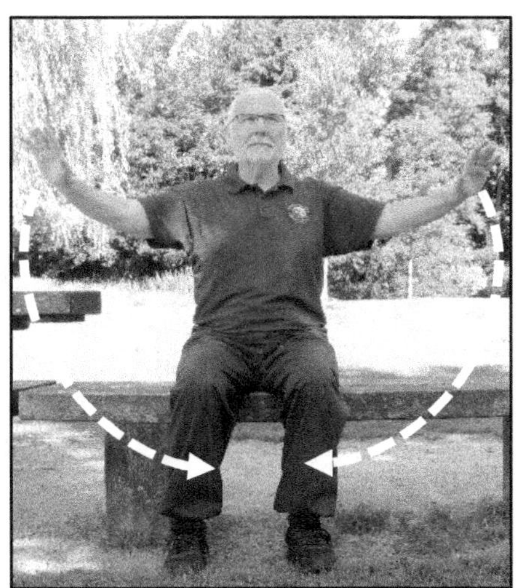
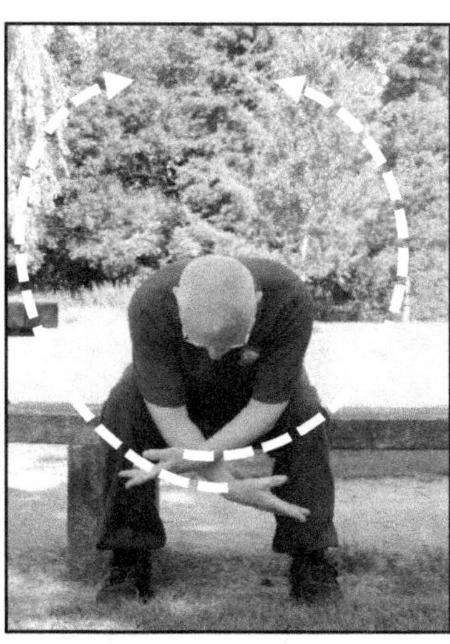

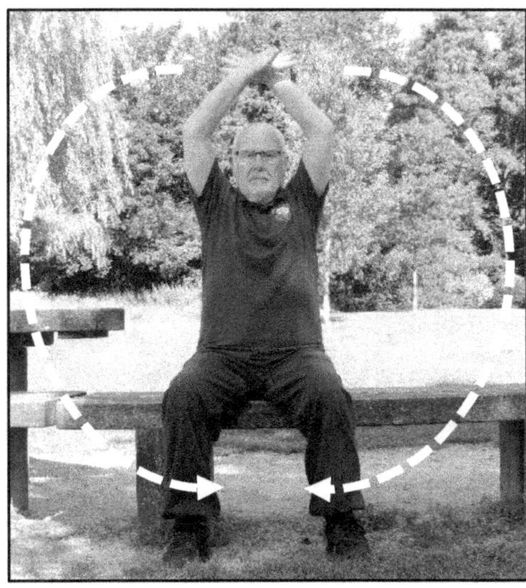

Lean forward and reach upwards only within your limitations and capabilities. Importantly, <u>stretch</u> upwards and <u>relax</u> downwards.

Posture 16. Rotating the Flywheel

From the final lowering of the previous posture, relax down and to the right, then continue relaxing as you sweep to the left and stretch up above your head or as high as you can. Continue circling as you relax down to the left. Then, "put the brakes on" and reverse the movement using the stored momentum. Perform this movement slowly and carefully to avoid dizziness. When you develop a certain amount of flexibility you might wish to add a slight turn of the waist to the sideward/upward movement. Initially, to avoid strained ribs muscles, be careful not to overstretch upwards.

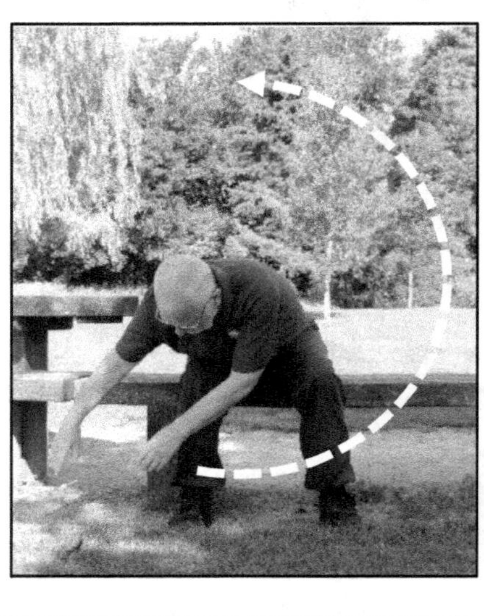
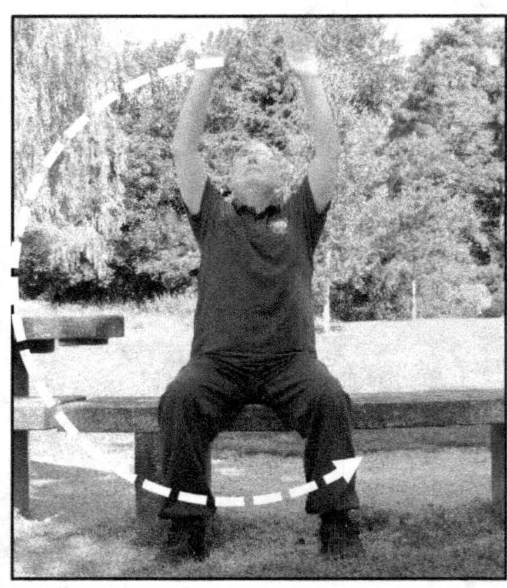

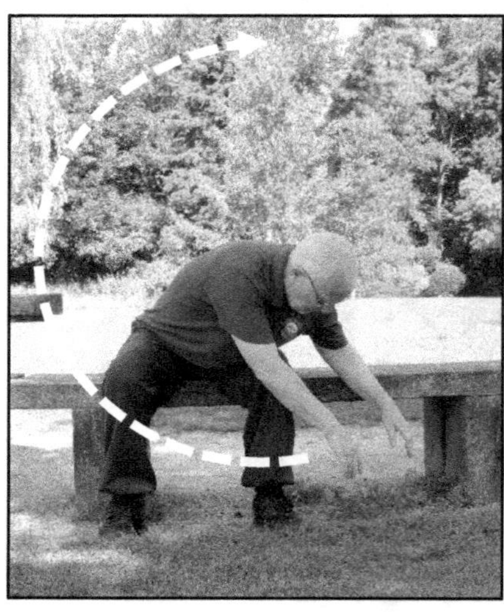
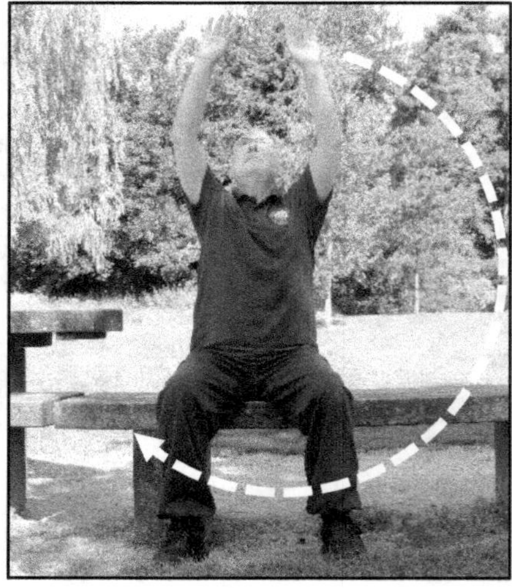

Posture 17. Bouncing the Ball While Marching

This adapted exercise is effective for helping to maintain and develop balance and coordination and aids concentration.

Bring your feet slightly closer together. Raise and lower the left arm as in *Regulate the Breathing* posture but a few times like bouncing a ball slowly and gracefully. Do this while the opposite knee is raised. Importantly, try to keep the raised knee still (there is a tendency to bounce the knee). Then, lower your foot gently, placing it back on the floor. Perform the movement on the opposite side.

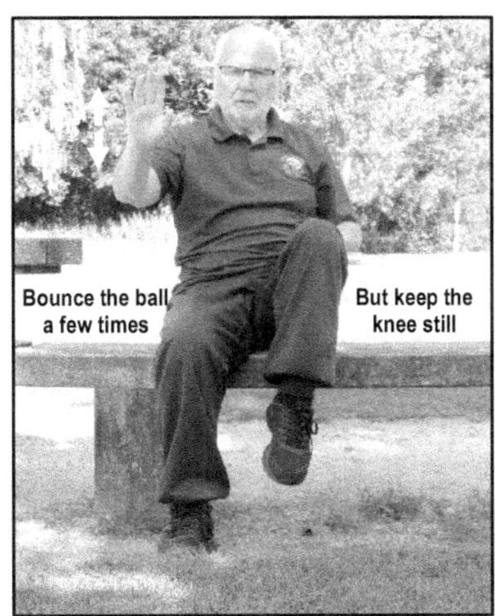

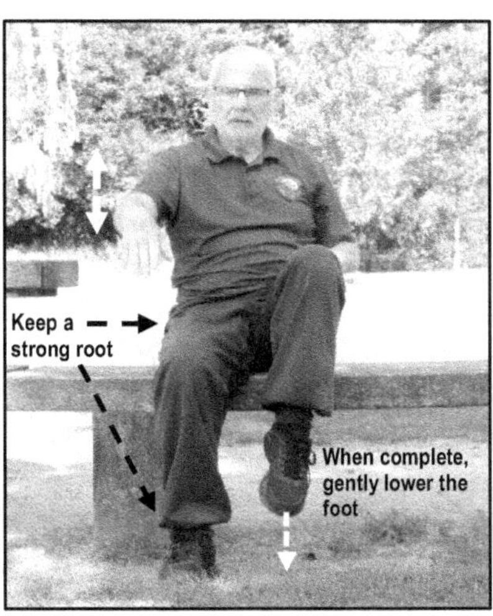

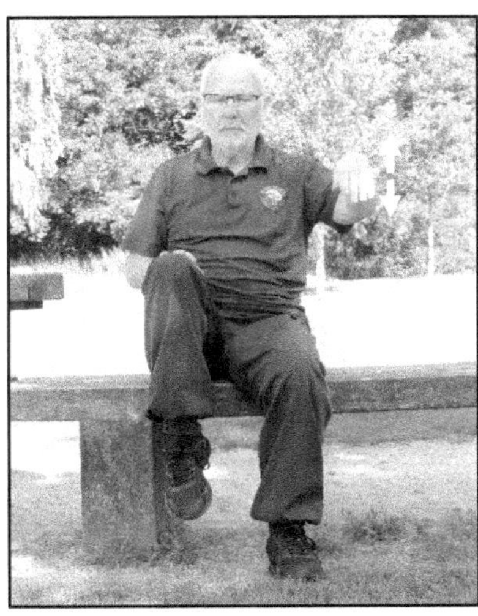

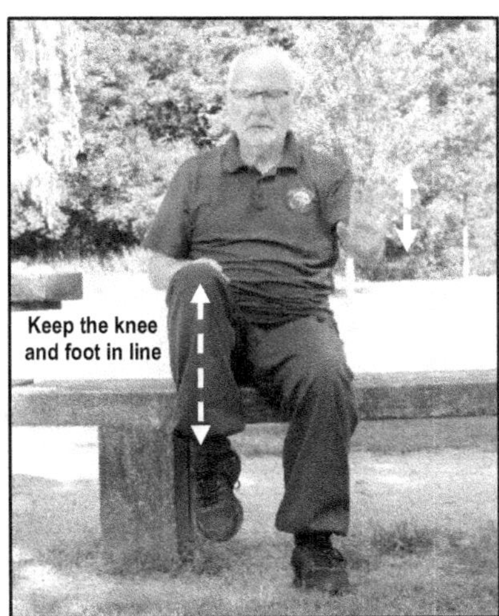

As there is a common tendency to raise the leg in a valgus (knock-kneed) manner with the foot everted (tilted outwards), try to ensure that you raise the knee up straight with the foot pointing slightly down and in line with the knee (as shown above).

Posture 18. Regulating the Chi

We began the form with *Regulating the Breath*. As we have now mobilised everything including our Chi, so it will now be flowing more actively and effectively, we now need to settle everything down so that the Chi and fluids continue to flow and function optimally and will not become scattered and dissipated. To this end, we must now *Regulate the Chi*.

Whether or not you believe in Chi flow etc., this posture has general beneficial physical and mental effects. For example, it is useful for calming the mind and breath and fully relaxing the body after the exercises. In Western terms we might think of it as a warming-down exercise. In Chi Gung, there are particular visualisation techniques for this posture with regard to Chinese medical theory, but this requires instruction from a teacher. Here it is best to just pay attention to the breath. Using a cleansing breath as we did at the start of the form, breathe-in as you lift your hands (as if using them to draw air into the lungs) and breath-out as you press the hands down (as if pressing down on the abdomen, which in turn pushes the air out of the lungs). You are not particularly active here, so do not overdo the deep breath as it might cause dizziness. Repeat a few times if you wish.

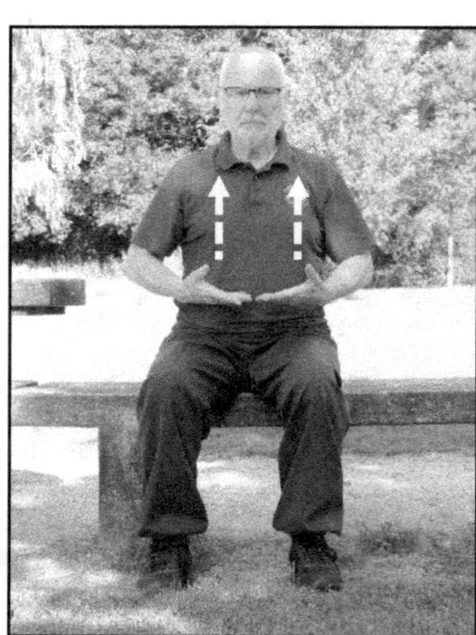
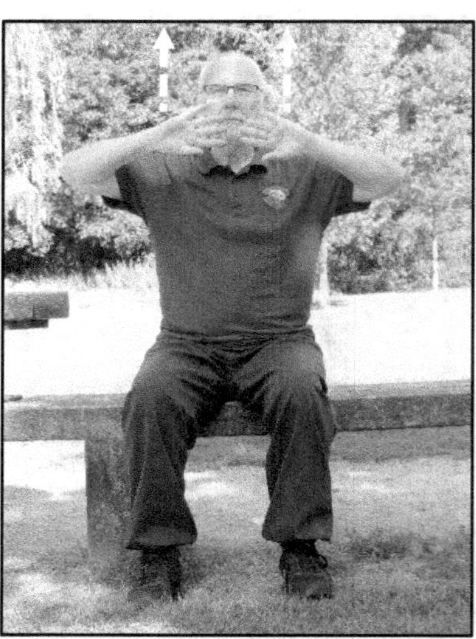

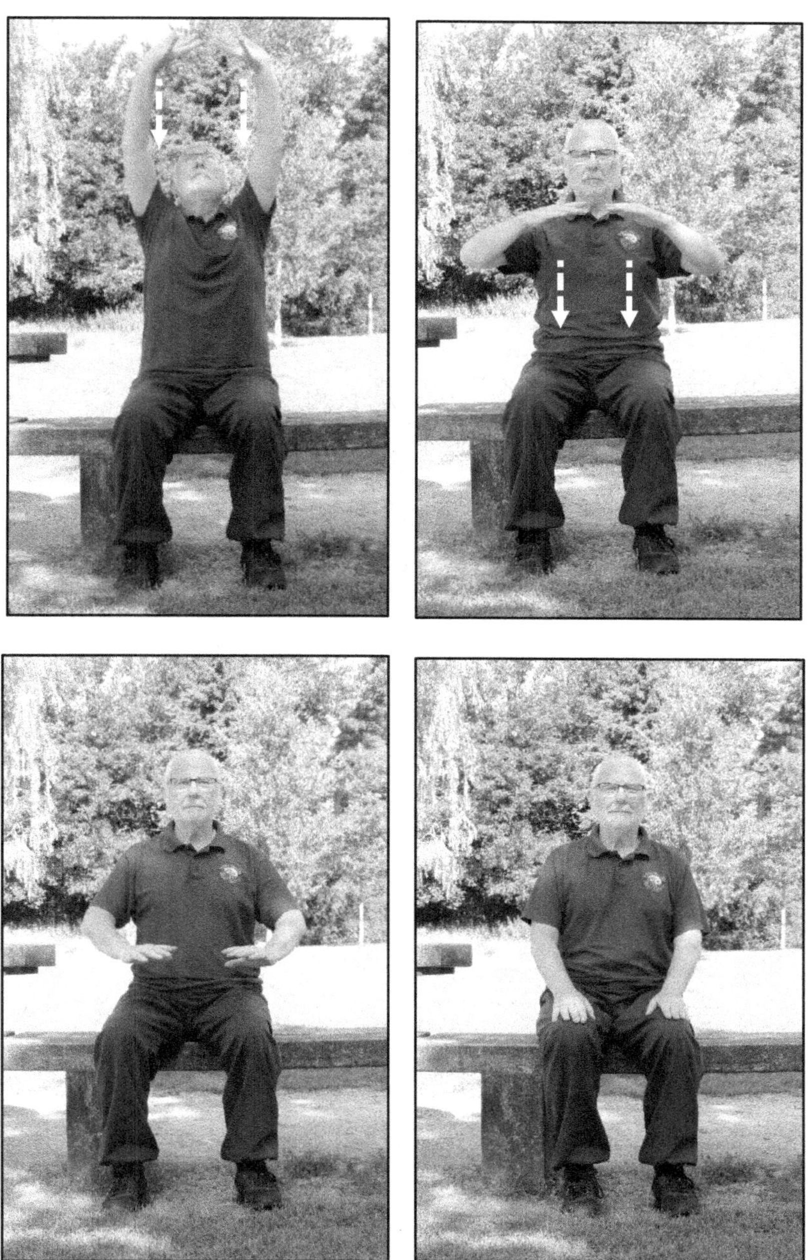

With a final in-breath, visualise the breath moving down to the *dantien* (just below the navel). At the same time, the hands are drawn in to rest at that point. Thus, you are closing in and settling everything down to your centre. Finally, let your breath calm to a natural relaxed state. Here you can either keep your attention at the *dantien* or on the calm breath moving in and out.

Note. It is best to use the same number of repetitions for each of the above postures, e.g., 1-3 to develop and practise a normal <u>regular</u> routine, 6-9 for the enthusiastic! ☺.

****

As with the previous set of exercises, these eighteen postures can be used as a stand-alone form. However, they are additionally effective if practiced after the mobilising and stretching exercises. Furthermore, practicing this form will also prepare you for practice of the slightly complex postures, transitions, and rhythmic nature of the more dynamic form of Chi Gung known as Tai Chi, which can be adapted for seated practice by a competent teacher.

5 SLOWING DOWN EXERCISE – TAI CHI

"To counter the unhealthy effects of the frantic pace of modern life, it is imperative that, in our free time, we try consciously to pause and slow down… slowing down is helpful in reducing mental and physical tension… Beyond the immediate effects of an exercise session, slowing down exercises influence the pace of the daily rhythm in what we do, how we talk and think"

Nyanaponika Mahathera

Without entering a discussion of the complexities and causes of anxiety, stress, and their relationship to the development of poor physical and mental health (See *Understanding Chi Kung* 2nd ed. for more detail on this topic), it would be safe to summarise that because of the "frantic pace of modern life" with all that it entails, we become further locked into unhealthy physical and emotional thought patterns and inappropriate physical action (or inaction). In order to counter this and the potential adverse effects on health and well-being, we need to set time aside each day to sooth our stress-filled mind and body and infuse it with calm. As Master John Farrell (2014) points out:

"This meditative aspect of Chi Kung engenders clarity of mind, calms the emotions and consequently, invigorates the spirit… helps to create a healthy, co-ordinated mind and body that is better able to deal with the pathogenic stressors, which individuals may encounter in their daily lives… enable the practitioner to relax the mind and body at deeper levels, assisting in the removal of more chronic or subtle tensions that may build up as a result of the increasing stress and pace of modern life."

Certainly, the previous exercises will help in this way if practised regularly and correctly but we can further enhance this by incorporating a method combining a more dynamic form of slowing down exercise with relaxation and mindfulness. To this end, and this applies to all meditative techniques, we need to provide a daily space in which we can break away from our usual busy-ness.

Learning Tai Chi

There are several popular systems of Tai Chi, and although they might vary in their characteristics, from a health point of view, their basic principles are the same. There are many useful books on Tai Chi and a few very good ones, e.g. *Complete Tai Chi Chuan* and other books by Dan Docherty; *Tai Chi Chuan Classical Yang Style: The Complete Form and Qigong* by Yang Jwing Ming; *Tai Chi, Health for Life* by Bruce Frantzis; *A Study of Taijiquan by Sun Lutang* translated by Tim Cartmell (See bibliography). However, there is no substitute for being taught by an authentic teacher but in the event of none being available, it is sometimes expedient and helpful to learn a simple form from a book or a video.

Relevant to this publication and for the purpose of a daily "slowing down exercise" as suggested by Nyanaponika Mahathera, I have provided a short but useful section of form, which should prove beneficial for individuals who wish to embark upon the further study of Tai Chi Chuan. Arguably, there is little point in providing a detailed description of a whole Tai Chi form in a book, as experience informs me that only learning it from a book can be a somewhat laborious task, which causes some potential enthusiasts to give up after a short while. As I mentioned, there is no substitute for an authentic teacher. However, the following postures provide a foundation for learning Tai Chi, and if you persevere in study, you will have a good basic slowing down exercise for daily use. Furthermore, you will find it much easier to learn a longer form when you locate a suitable Tai Chi teacher, i.e., once you have a general feel for the characteristic movement and postures you will feel less like a rabbit caught in headlights when newly joining a Tai Chi group, which can often discourage people from continuing. In addition, the nuances of movement in Tai Chi, such as found in Yang Chen Fu's 10 principles (Lo *et al*, 1985; Swain, 2005), when explained by a knowledgeable teacher, will be more accessible.

The form I am offering first, is the commencing or primary postures from *Sun Style Tai Chi* (see Appendix 1). I have chosen this first because it offers the usual beneficial weight-bearing and proprioception-developing postures of Tai Chi, without the slightly more difficult balancing required in the transitional steps of more commonly practised systems, which can sometimes result in pain and injury for the beginner who might have pre-existing joint/muscle/balance issues. A more commonly offered system is the popular *Yang Style Tai Chi* (see Appendix 2) with its more demanding stepping, so I have also included a useful section of the short Yang form for introduction and basic training in this new edition, which follows on from the presentation of the Sun style form.

Some notes on movement

"The movements are so slow and graceful" is a phrase often heard when an observer is describing their impression of someone performing Tai Chi. For observers and beginners, the graceful hand movements are often the focus of attention, which is why they might flail their arms around slowly with forced grace, attempting to imitate the hand movements and emulate the "ethereal" stillness of the Tai Chi teacher. Through correct instruction, beginners soon learn that the hand movements are only an expression of the energy derived from one's "root" or foundation - physical and mental, and the stillness is only a reflection of the confidence of that root.

The energy of the Tai Chi movement (and for that matter, Chi Gung) is generated from a profound mental and physical root, i.e., one is not distracted but aims to have mindful, one-pointed attention coordinating the purposeful movement of the limbs. The limbs move lightly and interdependently, yet maintain independence - as Chang San Feng advises, *"In motion all parts of the body must be light and nimble and strung together"*.

Primarily, the energy within any movement is generated, one might say triggered, from a stable mental root (itself more profound when one develops a stable physical root). The energy stored in one's centre or *dantien*, sinks into and engenders a stable, physical root. It is the source of the energy of the movement, which is then directed from the feet through the knees, through the hips, through the waist, spine, and shoulders, and is finally expressed in the hands. However, the energy that is expressed in the hands must be continually counterbalanced in the root: as Chan San Feng informs us, *"If there is an up there is a down…"* (Lo *et al*, 1985). One's energy movement is balanced within continual change and so is one's physical expression of that continual change, which is why the Tai Chi of a real master is so aesthetically pleasing as opposed to someone who just flaps their arms around in the air in exaggerated manner. Furthermore, when performing the movements, just as with Chi Gung postures, it is essential that the movements should be flowing, and relaxed but not flaccid, while postural alignment is maintained. Within each of the postures there should be a feeling of the body gently condensing and expanding or "opening and closing" from the centre or dantien.

To become familiar with this graceful and deceptively simple set of postures takes time, effort, and patience. But you should always keep in mind that developing effort and patience is just as much part of the mind-training of Tai Chi that slows things down, counters stress, and reduces *"the unhealthy effects of the frantic pace of modern life"*.

SUN STYLE TAI CHI

Posture 1. Wuji - No extremes / harmony

The Wuji or Wu Chi posture is basically the same as in the previous set, except that the foot position has the initialising characteristic of Xing Yi, the feet being angled at roughly 90°. Begin by relaxing (see appendix 5). Stand for a short while with your attention at the dantien before commencing the movements.

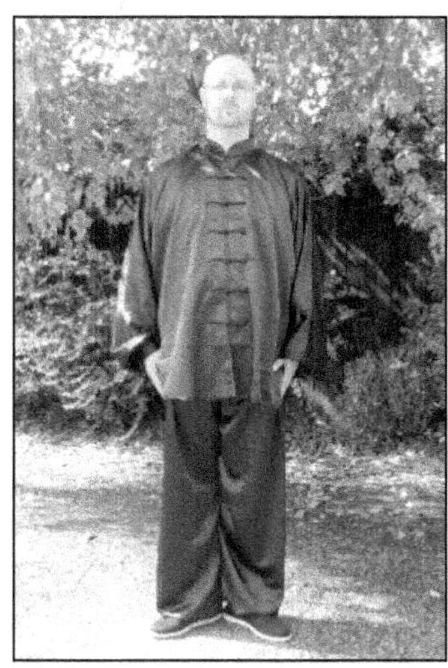

South
(As reference only for other postures)

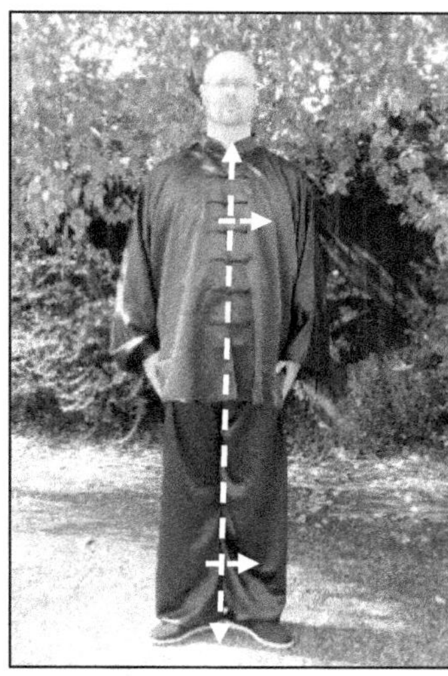

When moving the centre, try to avoid unintentionally lunging or rocking. To initiate the next posture, unlock the knees slightly in Wuji, this facilitates ease of movement.

Posture 2. Taiji - harmony within separation / change

1. Maintaining an upright posture, move your centre completely over to your left (see above photograph also).
2. Then, with the right foot, step slightly back to the rear of the left heel and place all you weight on the right side.
3. Turn your gaze to the Southeast and lift both hands up in that direction. The hands face each other but the left hand will be slightly more forward than the right because your torso is still facing slightly South as per Xing Yi form.
4. Sink onto the right leg. This sinking will create the energy to draw the hands down and in, as shown in the diagram.

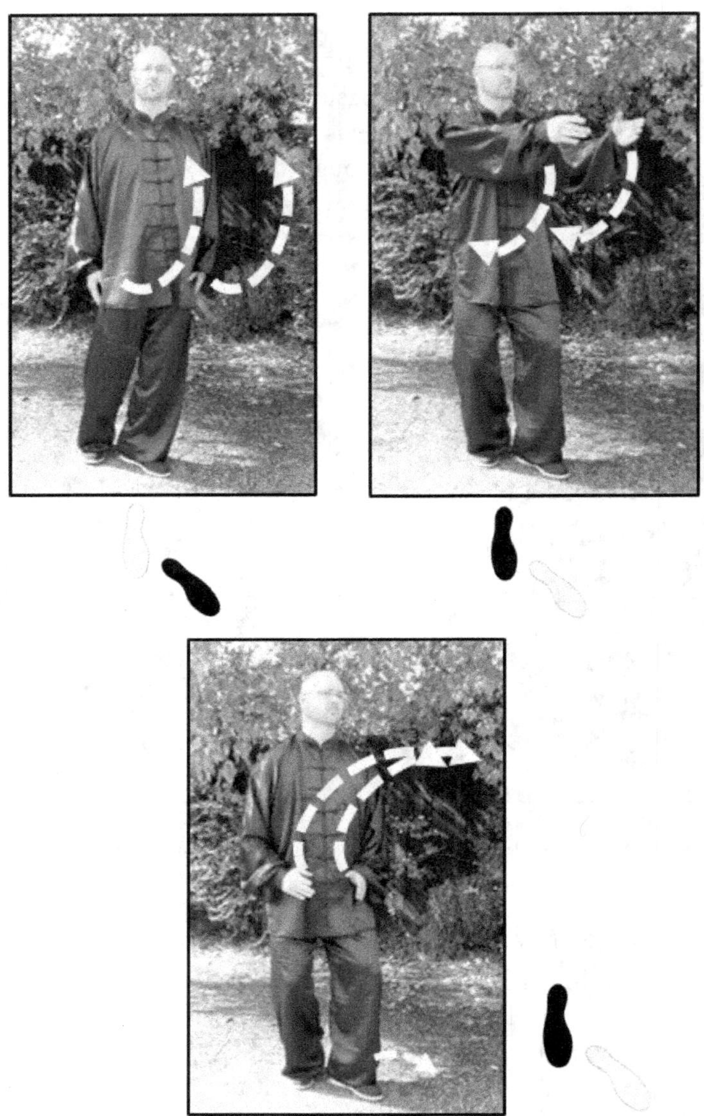

5. Draw the hands lightly up the torso, roughly to the level of the diaphragm, then step out on the heel of the left foot. This should be only to a distance that you could place the foot down flat without having to move your body forward.

6. Place the left foot down fully and shift your weight forward (about 70%). At the same time by pushing from the root of your right leg, extend the arms maintaining the slightly offset hand position to about the level of the upper chest/chin.

7. Push a little further and when nearly all your weight is on the left leg move the right foot slightly behind the left foot.

8. The left foot is now fully weighted, and the right foot is weighted only enough to stabilise your single-leg posture.

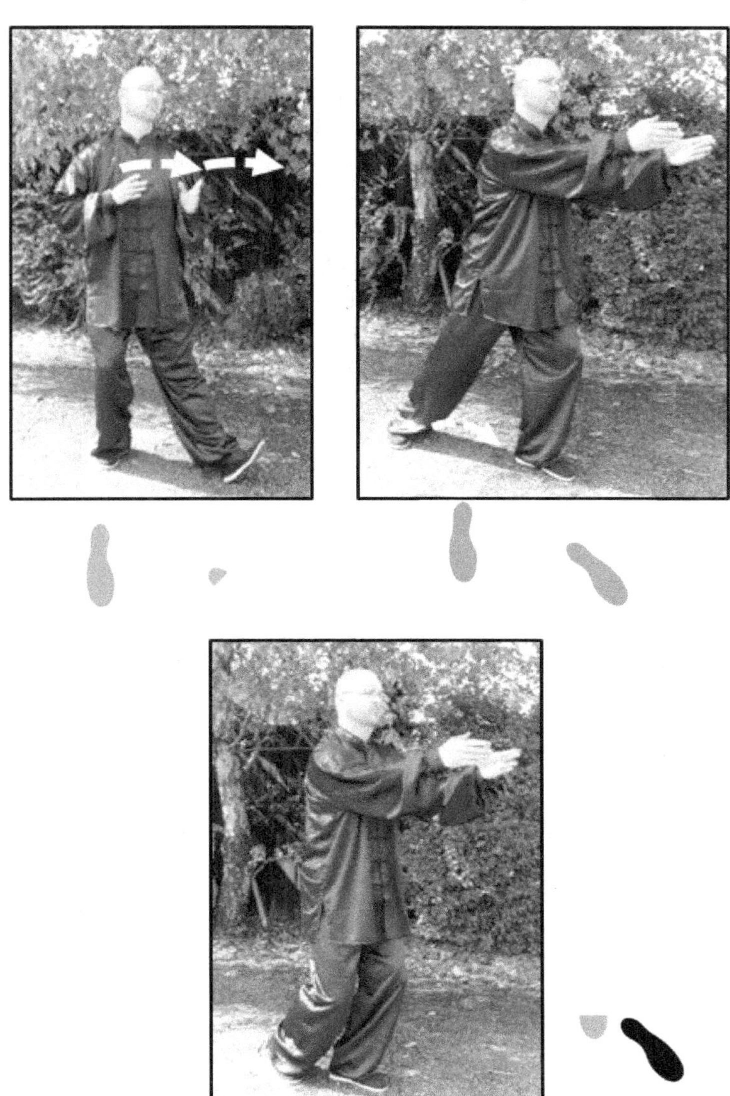

Posture 3. Lan zha yi - Lazily tying back the clothes

1. Shift all your weight back onto the right foot and step inwards with the left foot (more commonly this is done by pivoting on the heel). Place all your weight on the left foot ready to turn. *

    Turning, especially in martial arts is a precarious movement as we naturally lift our root in order to turn. Long story short, the twine-toed, knock-kneed posture, not only prevents undue torsion of the knee joint while turning but maintains one's root by driving it downward instead of losing it upward. Thus, a profound root is maintained while turning, ready for the next step.

2. As you begin this step, keeping the hands at the same level, turn the right palm upward and the left palm down. At first it is best to touch the right wrist with the left index finger and thumb. This helps to keep the hand positions correct.

3. The inward step of the left foot should cause your body and thus your hands to spiral to the Southwest (right). As you do this, place all your weight on the left foot to complete the turn. Now, raise your right heel so your foot can easily pivot on the ball into a natural position of a cat-posture, i.e., no weight on the foot, just the ball of the foot touching the floor.

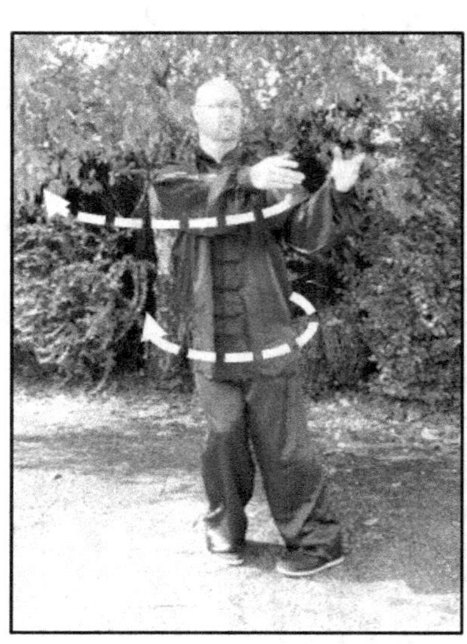
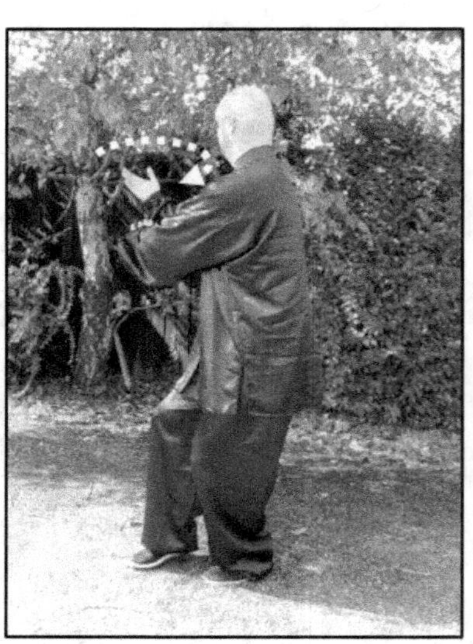

4. Using the spiralling energy of the waist-turn, continue to circle the palm to the right side and forward to brush near the cheek.
5. Then step out on to the heel of the right foot without having to move your body forward.

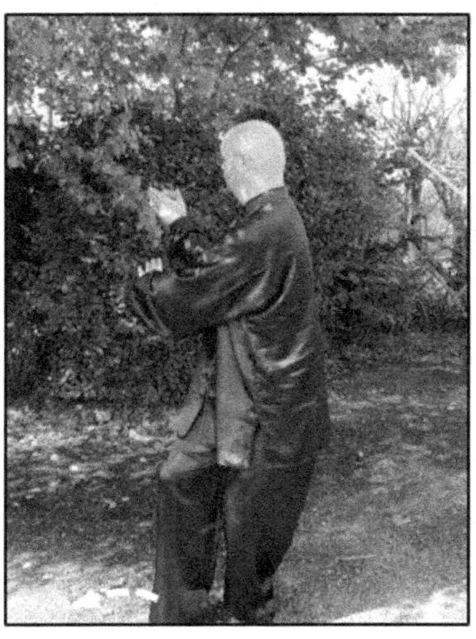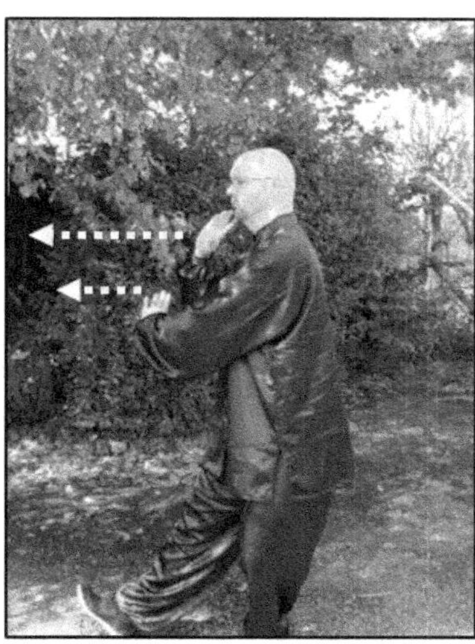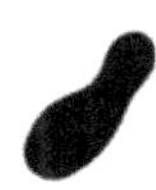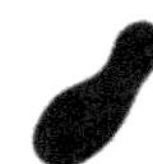

5. Place the right foot flat on the floor and from your root deliver 70% of your weight onto the right leg. As you do so, push both palms forward, the left slightly behind the right.
6. Without leaning and when your palms have reached the full extension (without locking your elbows) and all your weight is committed to the right leg, move the left foot next to and slightly behind the right foot. Most of your weight is now on the right foot.
7. You should be strongly rooted on the right foot with the feeling that you could spring forward from the left foot or easily return to stepping backwards with the left foot.

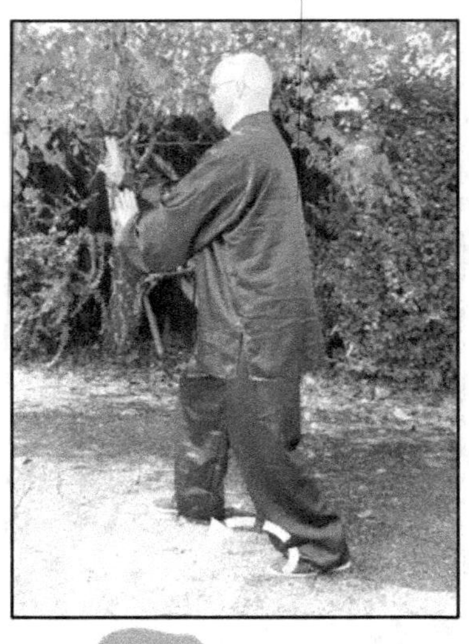 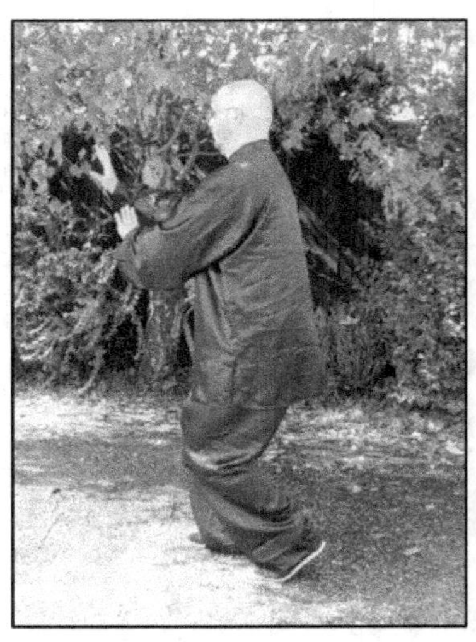

Posture 4. Kai shou - Open

Now you will turn back facing South.

1. Turn the left foot inwards and down so that the foot is pointing South. Shift your centre completely to the left foot.
2. Turn the right foot in (more commonly this is done by pivoting on the heel) so that it is also points South, this will cause your torso and arms to spiral South also.
3. Just as you face south, the palms should now be facing each other, and all your weight should transfer to the right leg – although visually, the stance should appear double-weighted.
4. Open the palms to shoulder width, the thumbs will be roughly in line with the shoulders.

Although one should not worry about coordinating the breath with the postures at this stage without instruction, it is useful and relaxing at this juncture in the form to take a "cleansing breath", breathing in as you *open*.

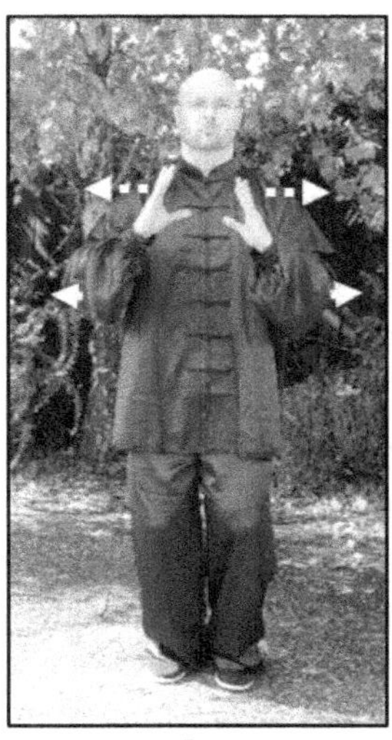 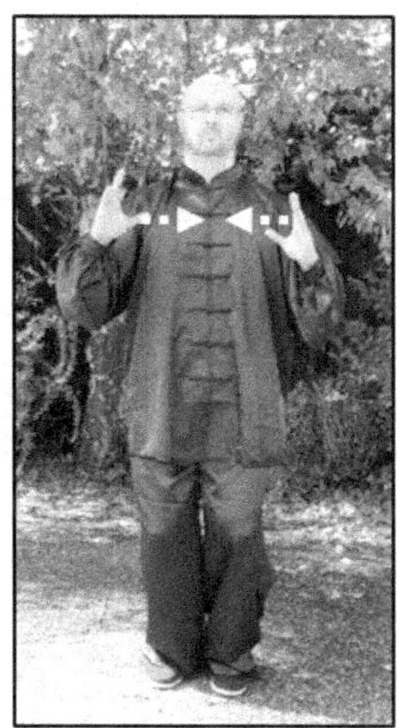

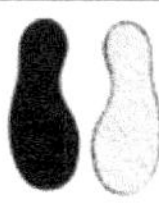

When you become more familiar with the form, the "opening" begins as you start to turn South.

5. He shou - Close

From *open* gently push the palms closer together, thumbs about one inch apart.

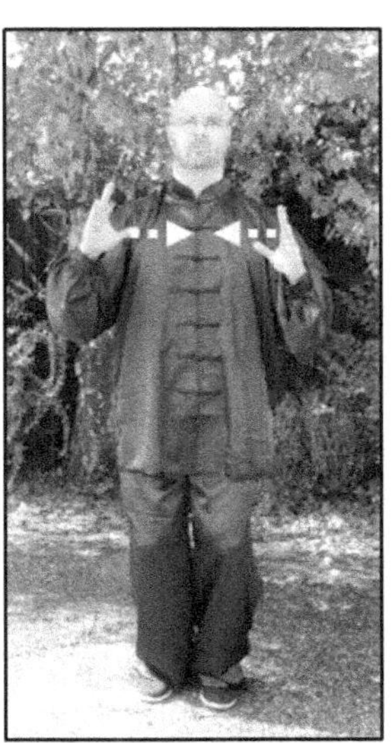 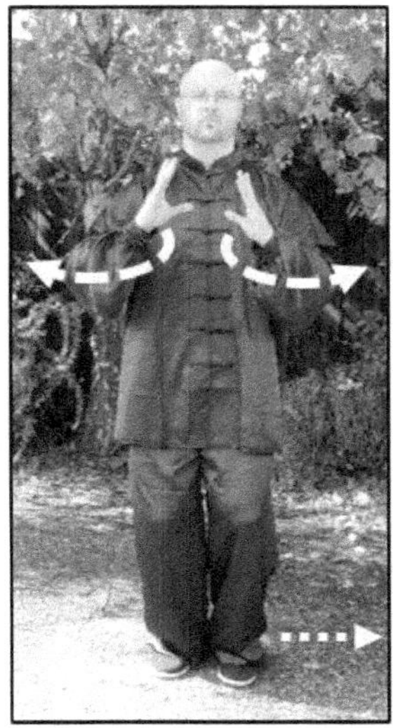

To reiterate, one should not worry about coordinating the breath with the postures at this stage without instruction, but it is useful and relaxing at this juncture in the form to take a "cleansing breath", having breathed in as you *open*, now and breathe out as you *close*. Try to feel a gentle expanding and condensing of the whole body.

Posture 6. Dan Bien - Single whip

Still facing South, you will step out and push the palms forward and out in the direction of the arrows shown in the diagram above.

1. Looking on the right diagonal, step out to the left as far as you can to place your heel down without having to rock your body.
2. As you shift your body into a horse-riding transitional position push the palms forward slightlty and out to front and side.
3. Complete the movement by shifting some more of your weight to the left leg (70:30/60:40 - ish). Keep both legs bent with the left foot pointing to the corner.

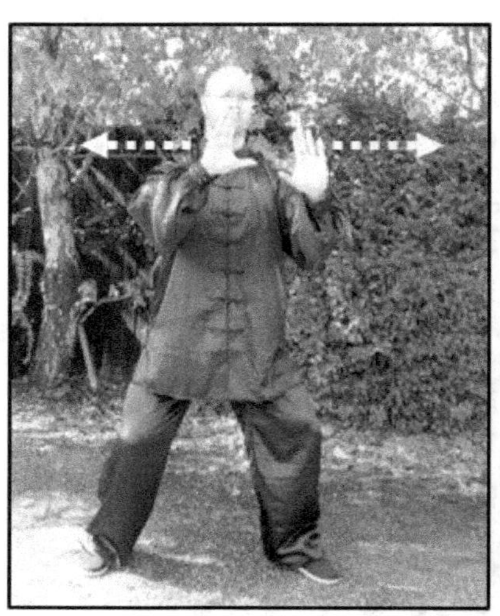
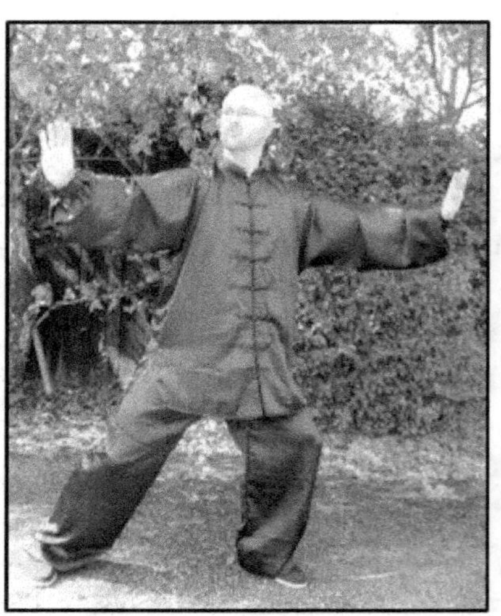

Posture 7. Yin Yang hun yi - Uniting yin and yang

This closing posture is a simplified adaptation of the closing posture of the complete form.

1. From single whip, sweep the hands in an arc to crossed, inward-facing fists.

2. At the same time, shift your weight onto the right leg and step in with your left leg to the original starting position.

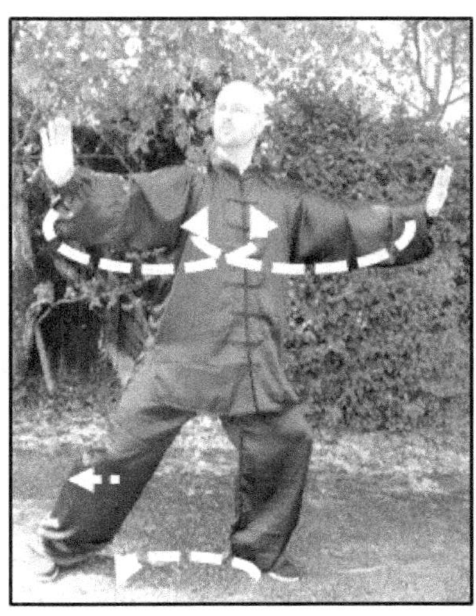

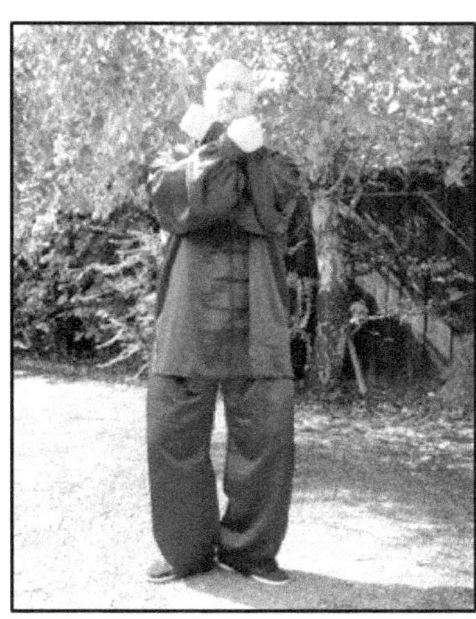

Posture 8. Wu ji huan yuan - Return to Wu Chi
1. Open the fists and sweep the hands down in an arc to the original position as you straighten the legs.
2. Finish with a cleansing/relaxing breath and return your attention to the dantien. Stand for a comfortable length of time as you settle and relax.

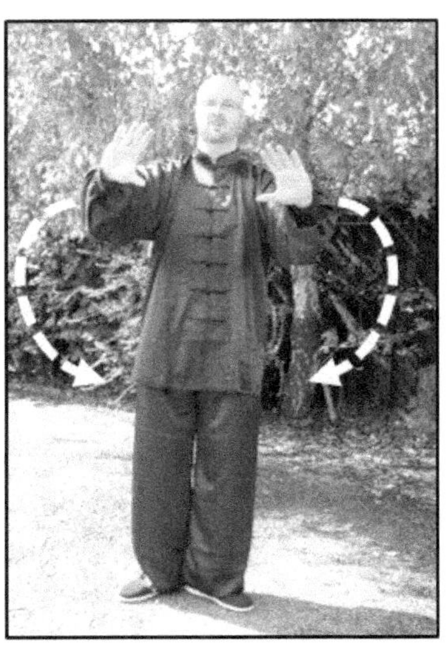

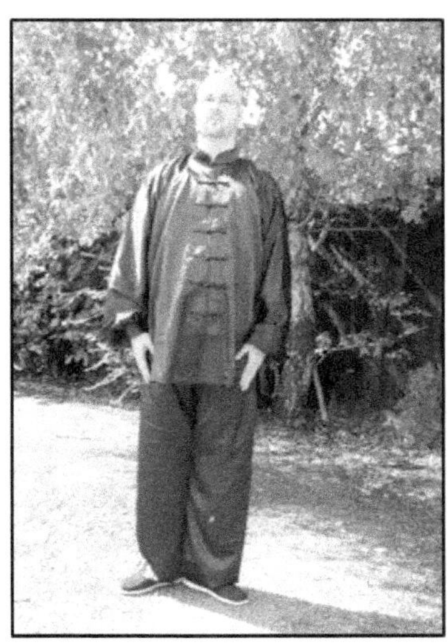

Practise the movements on a regular basis until you become familiar with the form. When competent, it is useful to extend the form by repeating the postures or if you feel adventurous, repeat in the opposite direction. The following chart shows the complete set in the opposite direction. However, the chart might also prove useful as a mirror image to aid learning the above.

The gentle focus and attention on root and movement within the form requires some degree of effort and practise, although this is not a rigid mental attention or control as one should also have awareness of the environment. It might be said that one should be mindful of the movement and as such one is mindful of each present moment of the movement. Thus, "...*the energy of the mind is not scattered, but focused and concentrated...*" (See Appendix 6. for a brief outline of mindfulness in movement).

SHORT SECTION OF THE SUN STYLE FORM
(Mirror image)

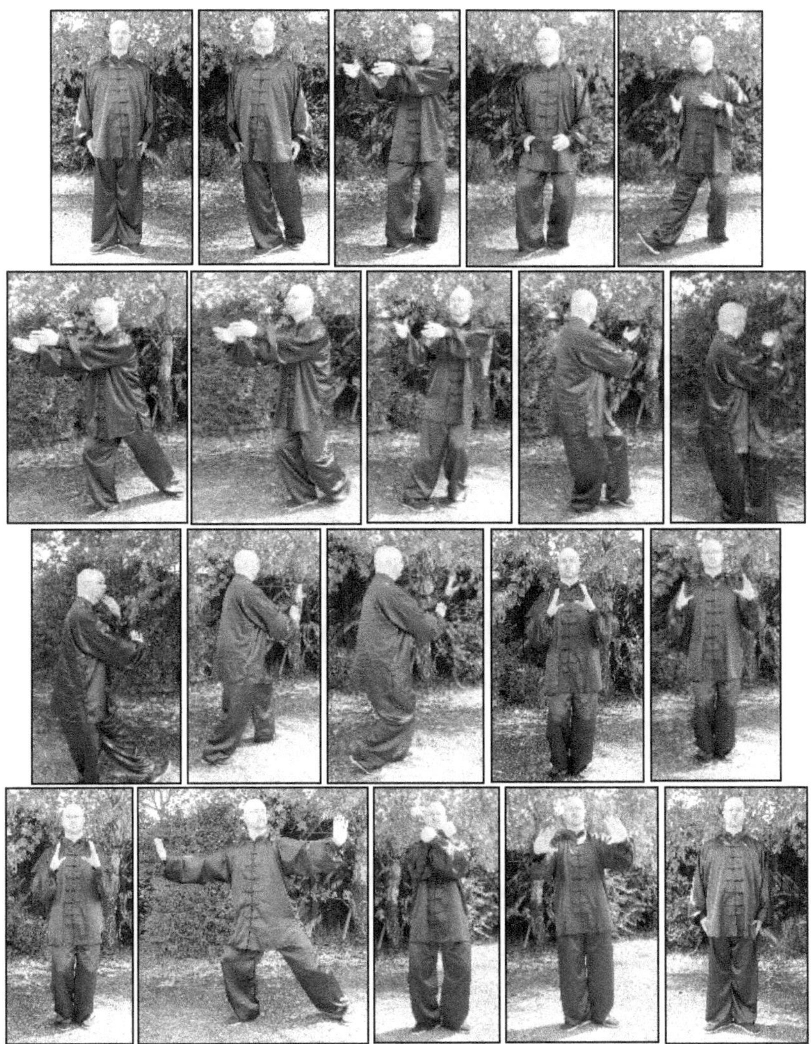

If you are interested in extending your study of this form you can find Sun Lutang's detailed explanation of the whole form in *A Study of Taijiquan* translated by Tim Cartmell (2003)

YANG STYLE TAI CHI

Posture 1. Yubei shi - Preparation (aka Wuji or Wu Chi)

The Wu Chi posture is basically the same as in Shibashi with correct spinal curves and postural alignment.

Although the legs are upright, the knees are slightly soft and unlocked.

Begin by relaxing (See appendix 5). Stand for a short while with your attention at the dantien. When you are ready, step out to shoulder width to commence Posture 2.

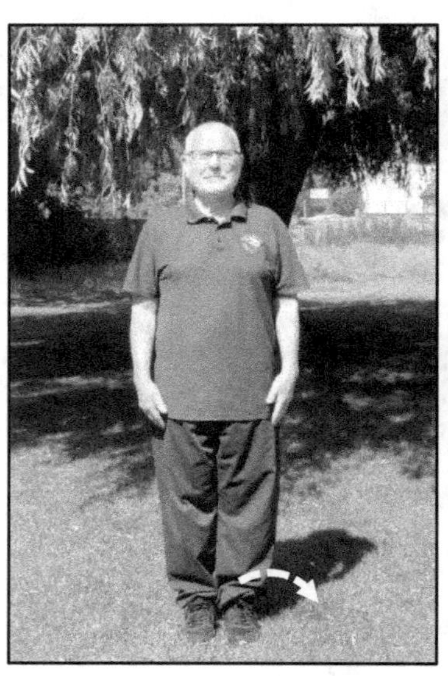 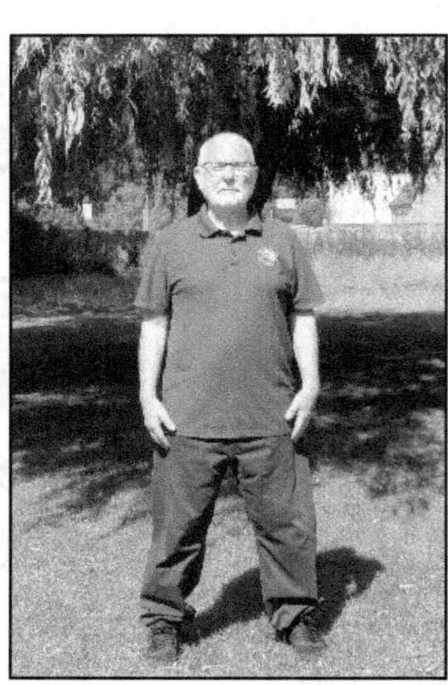

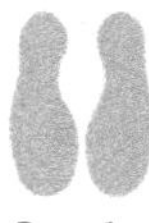

South

Posture 2. Qishi - Commencing (aka Taiji)

1. Shift your centre (weight) to the right foot without tilting or rocking.
2. Step a shoulder-width to the left, feet parallel, as above.
3. Without rocking, return to a central weight distribution.
4. Sink gently into the horse-riding posture.
5. Without tension, allow the arms to arc upwards and slightly in before brushing them down to resting level as shown in the photograph.

6. As the arms raise allow your body to rise and as they lower, sink into the horse-riding posture.

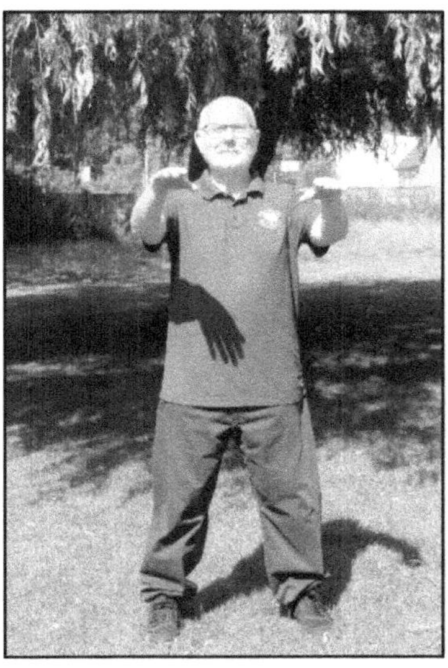 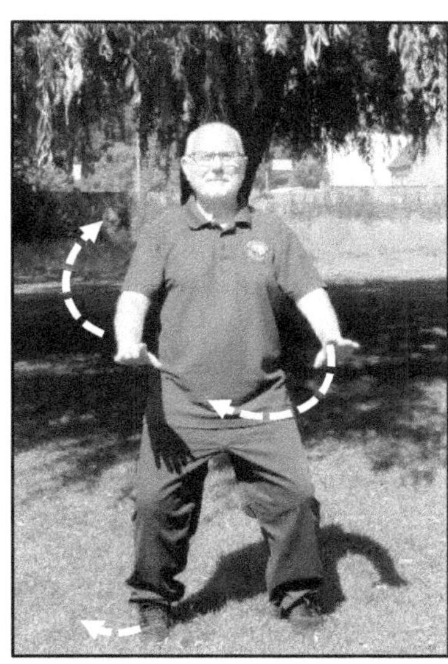

Posture 3.   (Peng Zuo) - Left Ward Off*

1. Move the centre to the left leg as and pivot on the right heel as you turn right (West). Begin to circle the hands as shown below.
2. Shift your weight to the right leg and begin to turn south.

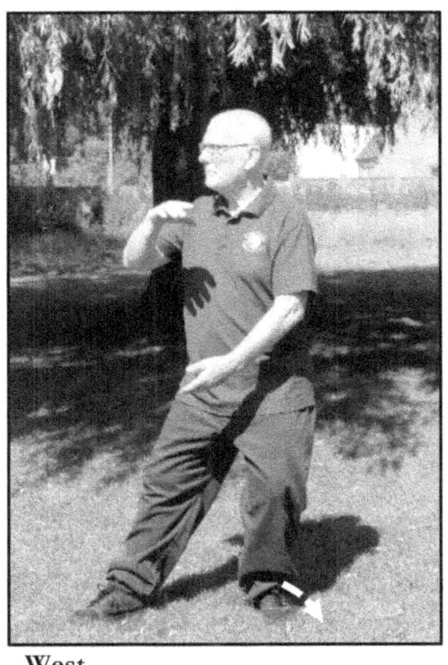

West

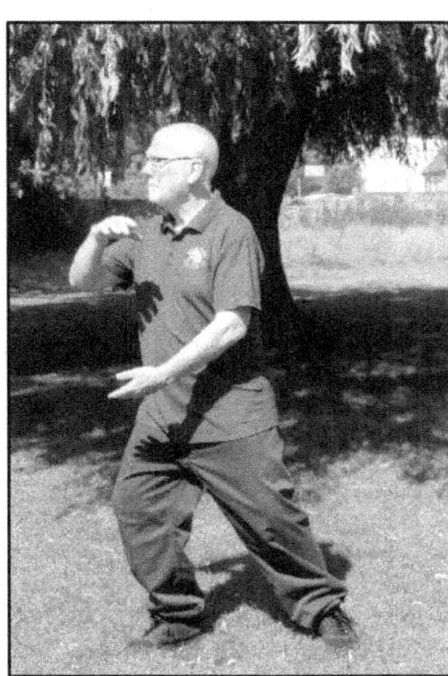

South

3. Step south by raising the left heel and placing it down again to step southwards.

4. Lower the ball of your foot and Move 70% of your weight on to the left leg, which is bent, 30% on the rear which is softly bent (*Bow Posture*).

5. As you move your weight forward raise the left hand to just below chin level as shown below, the emphasis of movement being on the forearm. The right hand brushes and presses down.

6. As you ward off to the left (South), the right toes pivot slightly inwards.

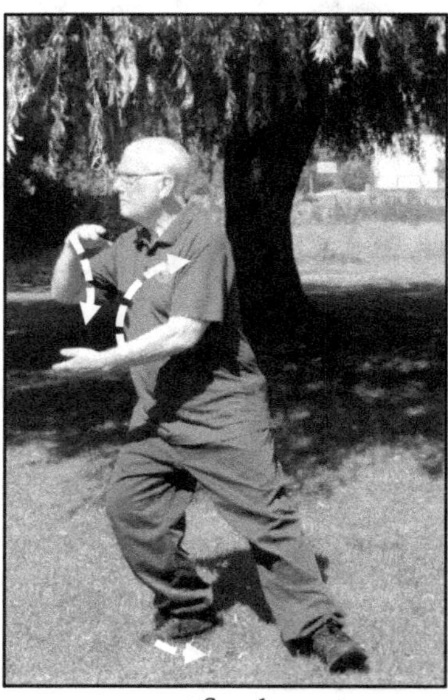

South

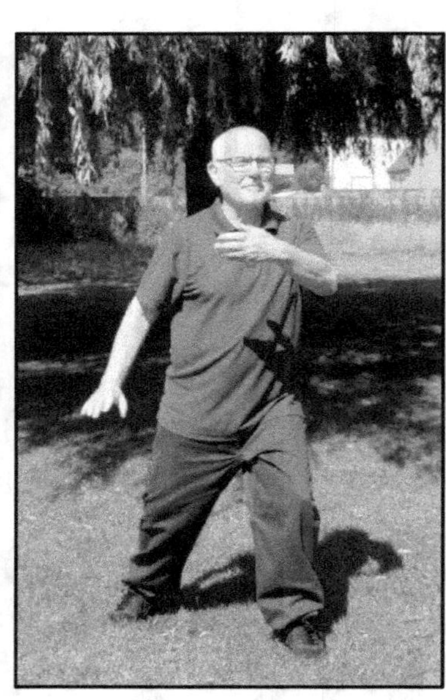

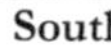

Posture 4. (Peng You) - Right (double)Ward Off *

1. Move the centre to the left leg and pivot on the right toes toward the right (West).

2. Rock the right foot and place the heel slightly forward.

3. Place the foot down and move 70% of the weight forward onto the right leg. Finally, pivot the left toes slightly inward.

4. The right hand curves up to ward off just below or level with the chin. At the same time the left palm curves forward just

behind the right palm. Like holding a small ball.

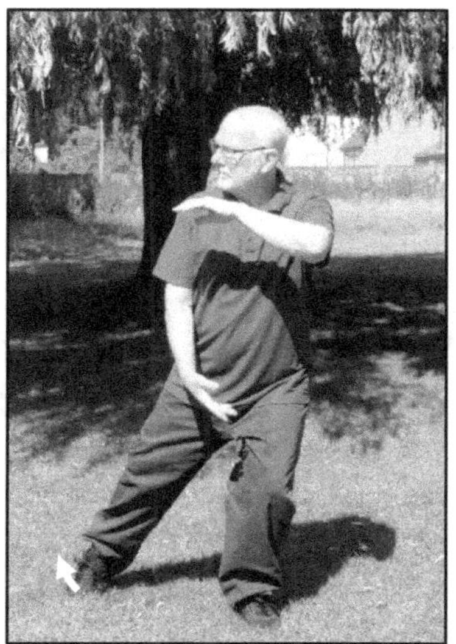 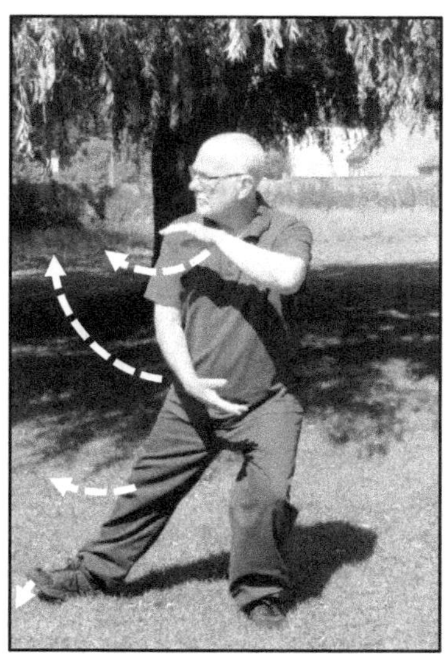

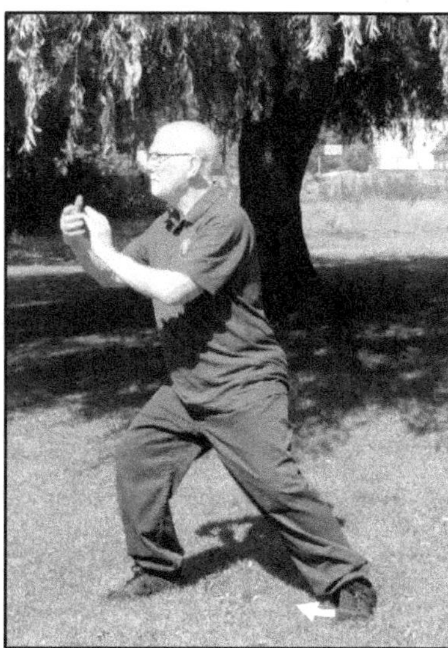

West

Posture 5. *Lu* – Rollback*

1. Turn your waist slightly right as you sweep both hands around and slightly diagonally, so the left palm faces up toward the right.
2. Move about 60% of your weight back to the left leg and as you turn your waist left, draw the palms down to the left. Keep the

left knee aligned with the right foot to avoid undue pressure on the joint.

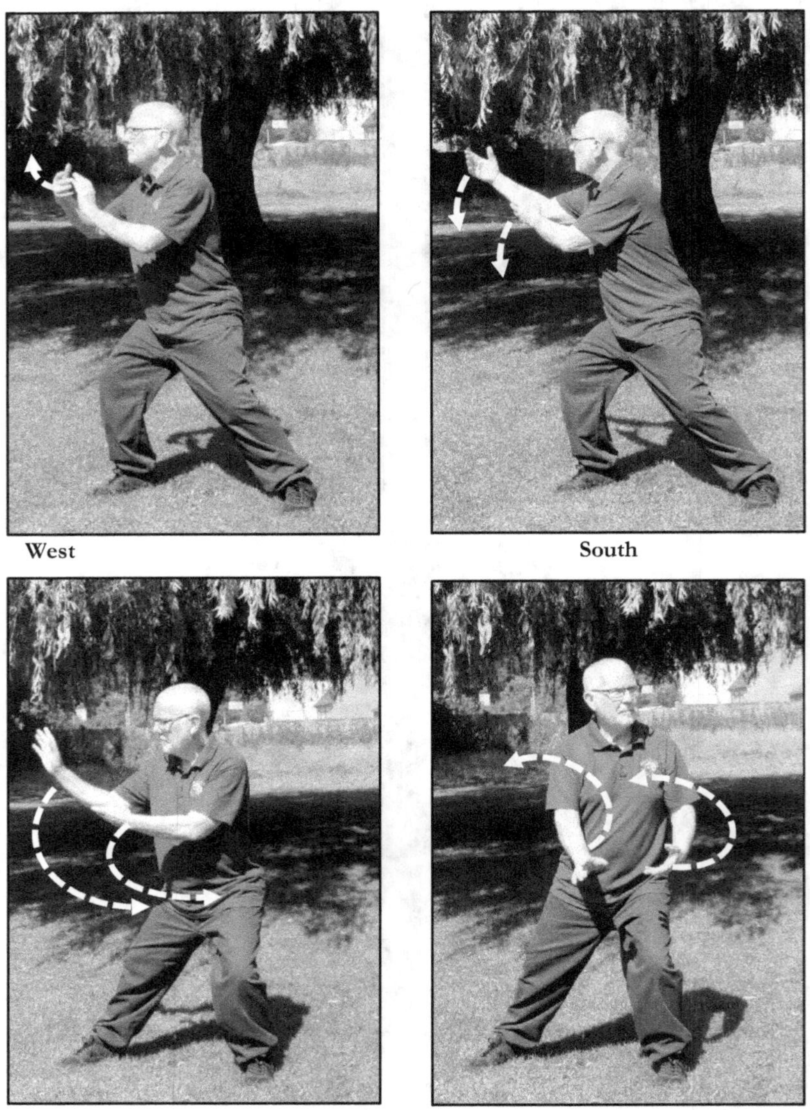

Posture 6. Ji – Press/Squeeze*
1. Continue circling the left palm up and forward.
2. At the same time, the right hand circles up back to ward off.
3. The left hand presses the right palm at or near the wrist.

106

4. 70% of your weight shifts forward into the bow posture and the palms move forward.

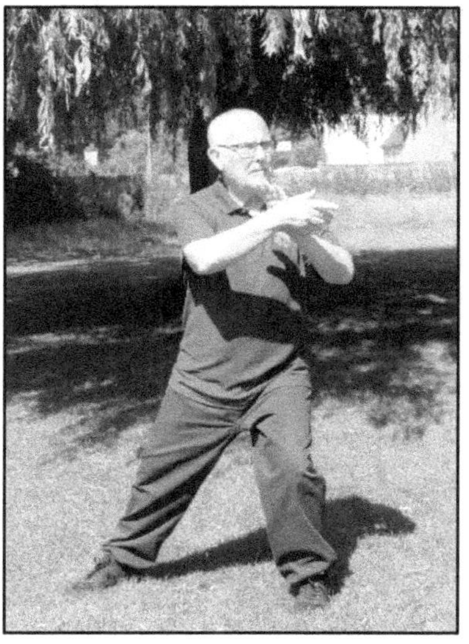
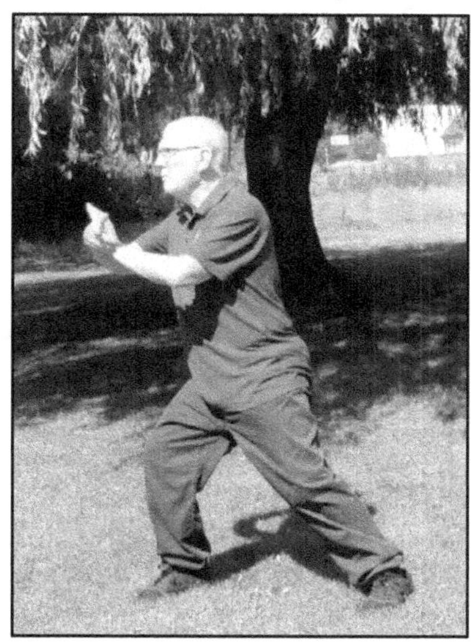

Posture 7. An – Push*
1. Cross the hands flat (left over right) and as you rock back sweep the palms out and down as you drop the elbows.
2. Move the weight forward. Settle the wrist and push the palms.

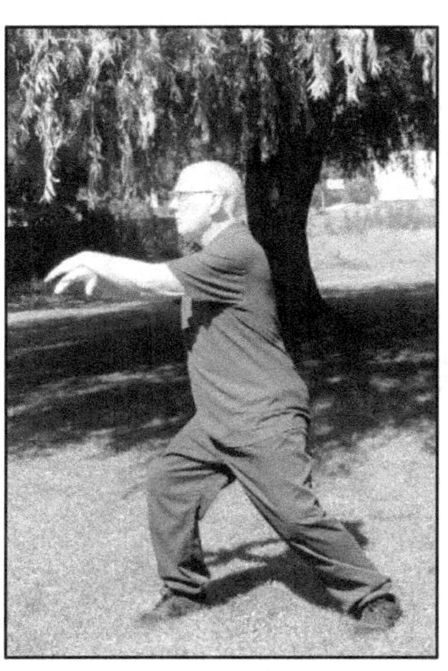
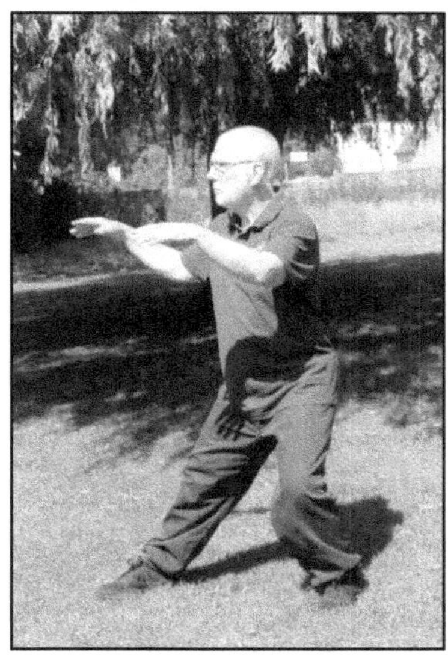

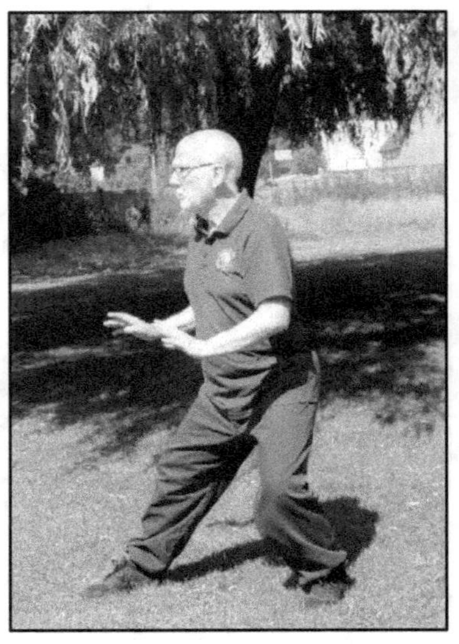 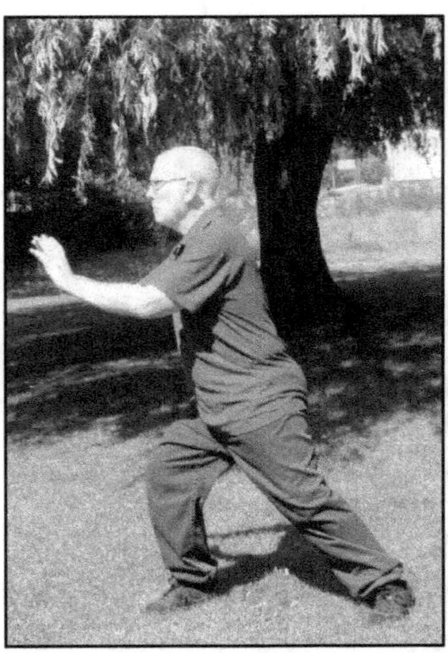

Posture 8. Dan Bien - Single Whip

1. Shift most of the weight to the left and twist at the waist to the left (East). The spiralling energy draws the hands across the body to the left.

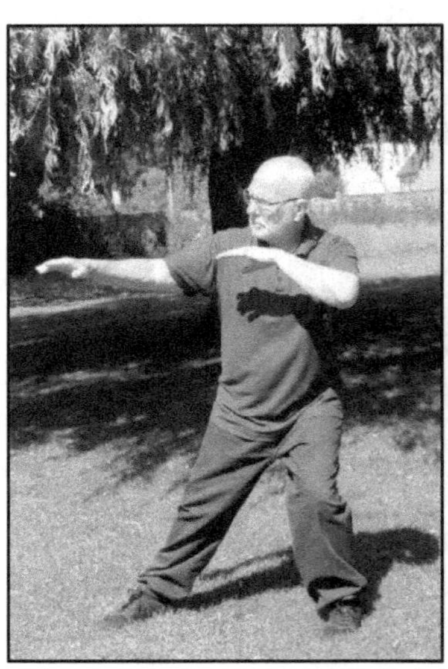 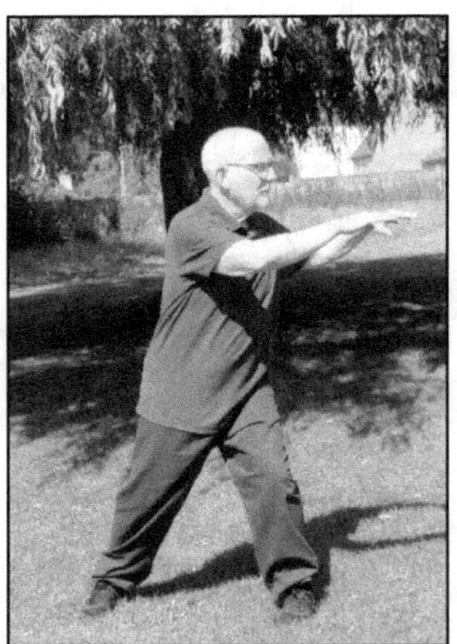

East

2. Shift 60% of your weight back to the right leg and twist your waist back to the right. The spiralling energy draws the hands across the body to the right. Pivot the right toe forward (South)

3. Squeeze the fingers and thumb of the left hand (Crane's beak) as shown in the photograph below

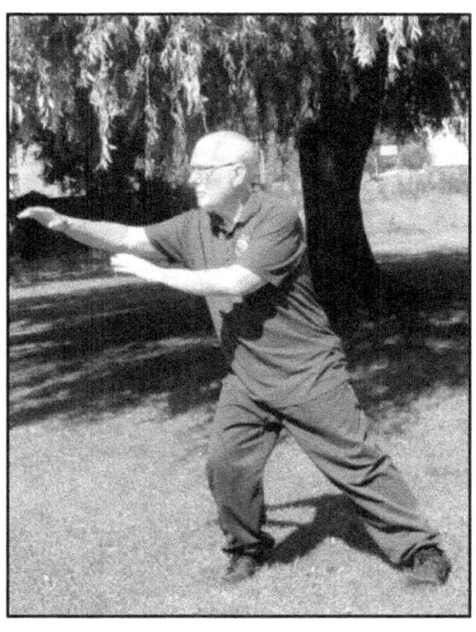 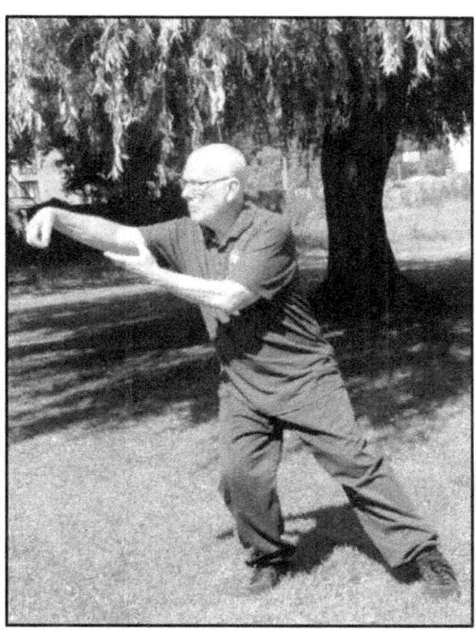

4. Move the left foot forward and left towards the Northeast
5. Move 70% of the weight to the left leg. Simultaneously sweep the left palm in an arc to the left (East).
6. Pivot the right toes in slightly.

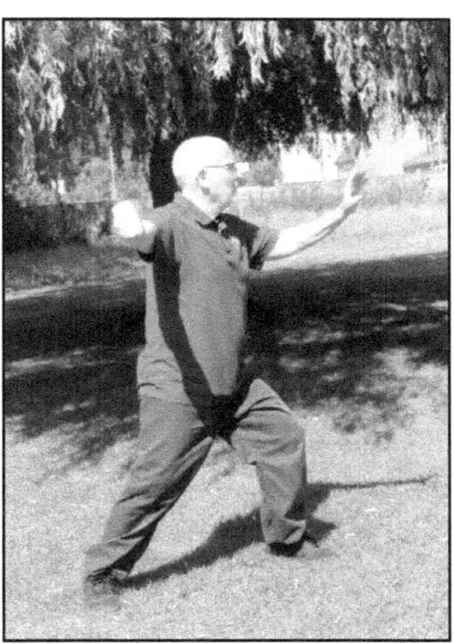 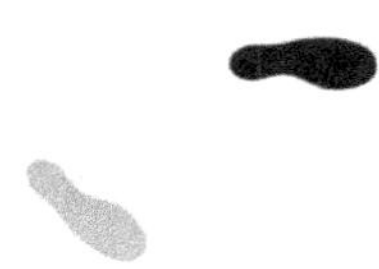

Posture 9. Shih Tzu Shou - Cross Hands

1. Move all your weight back to the right foot and as you turn right (South) sweep the right palm out to the right.
2. Sweep both palms down and up to cross at the chest, right hand outermost. Simultaneously, step with the left foot to *Mabu*.

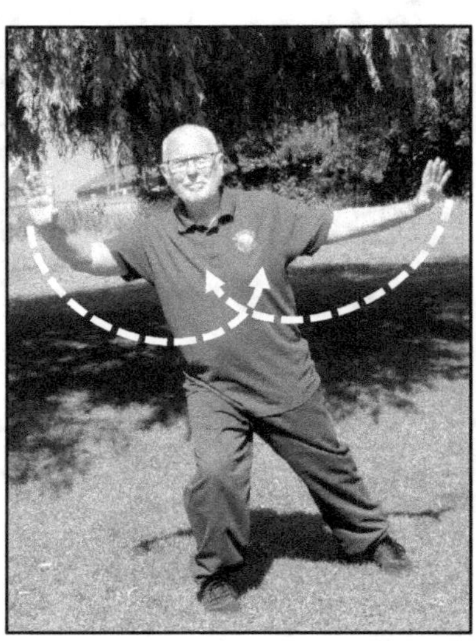
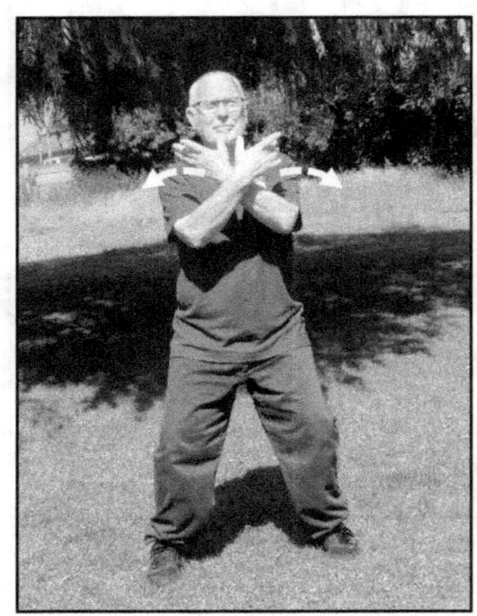

Posture 10. Shoushi - Closing (aka Return to Wu Chi)

1. Turn the palms flat (left over right) and sweep them out to shoulder-width.

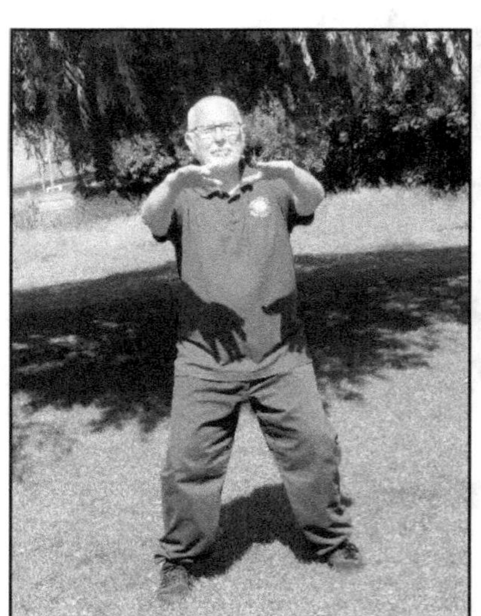
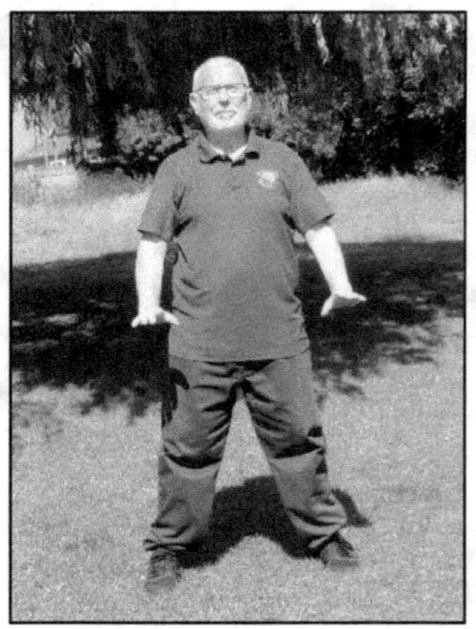

2. Brush them down to resting position. Place them on the side of the thighs.
3. Step in with the right foot next to the right.

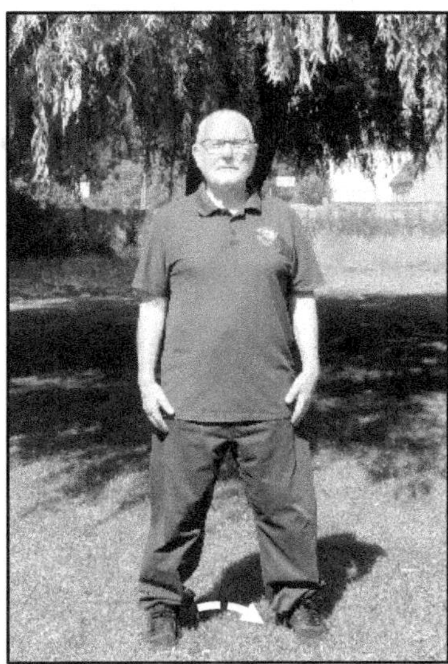 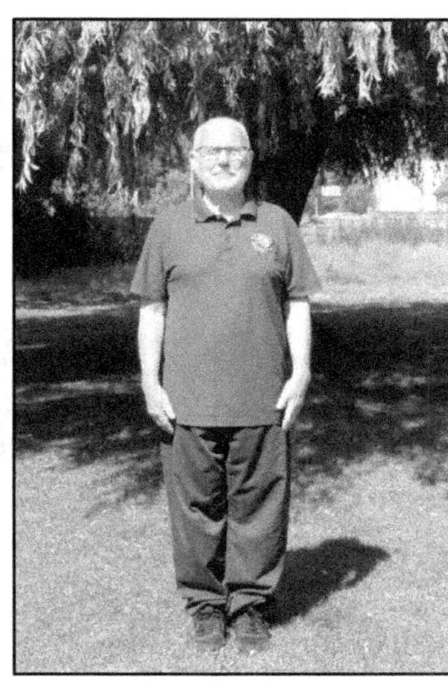

*Postures 3-7 are known **as** *Lan Qie Wai* or *Grasp the Sparrow's Tail*. They are 4 of the 13 basic postures of Tai Chi, i.e., 8 basic hand positions and 5 ways of stepping. One might say that these 4 forms, *Peng, Lu, Ji, An*, form the basis of martial application, the others being elaborations: *Tsai* -pull down; *Lieh*-split; *Zhuo*-elbow; *Kou*-shoulder. These, along with basic steps, *Jin*-forward; *Tui*-backward; *Ku*-dodging left; *Pan*-dodging right; *Ding*-central root, form the 13 basic postures.

Whatever System you focus on, practise the movements on a regular basis until you become familiar with the form. When competent, it is useful to extend the form by repeating the postures or if you feel adventurous, repeat in the opposite direction. The following chart shows the complete set in the opposite direction. However, the chart might also prove useful as a mirror image to aid learning the above.

Remember to apply mindfulness to the movement; you should try to be aware of each present moment of the movement. Thus, "*...the energy of the mind is not scattered, but focused and concentrated...*" (see Appendix 4. for a brief outline of mindfulness in movement).

SHORT SECTION OF THE YANG STYLE FORM
(Mirror image)

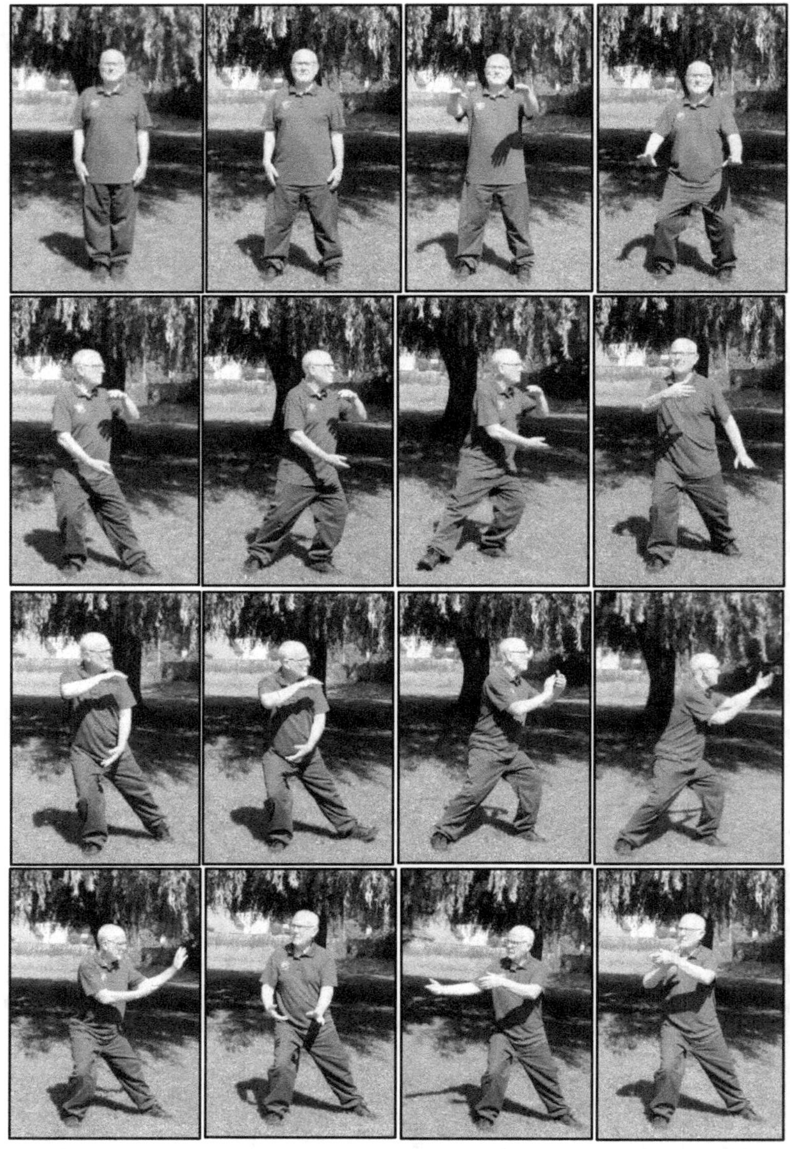

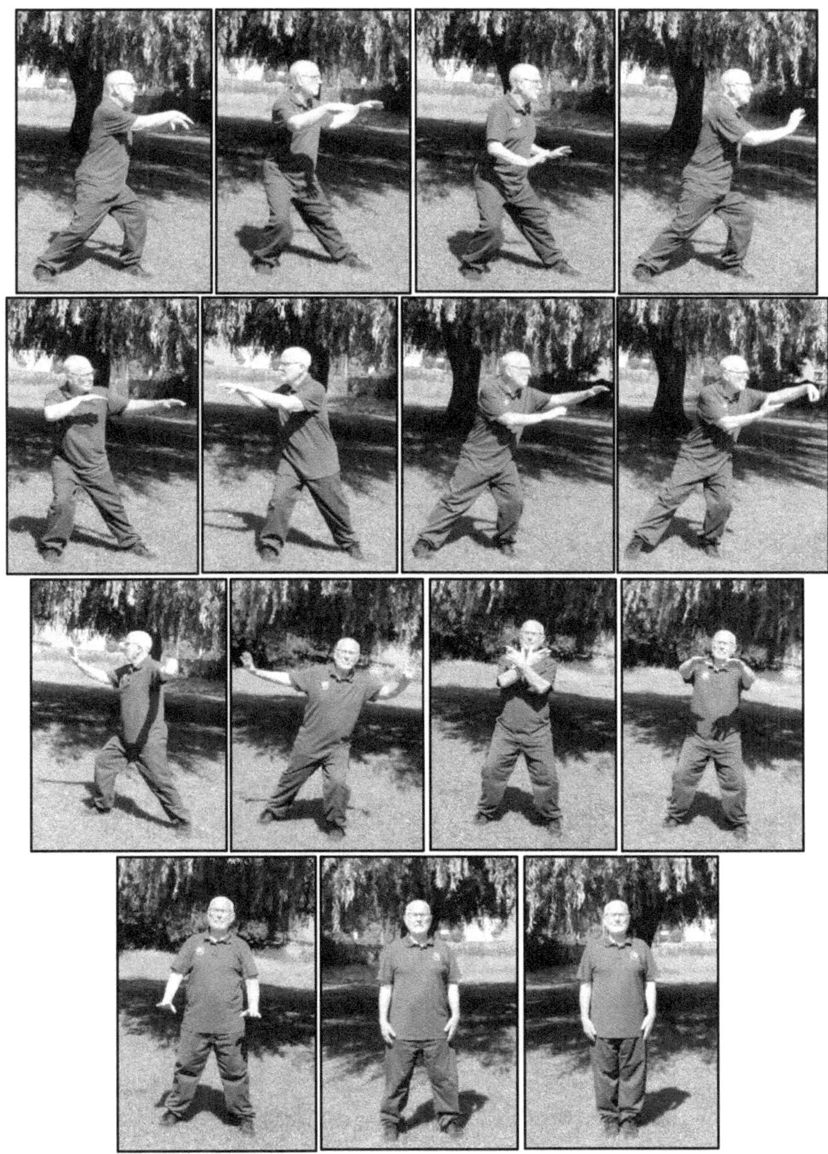

If you are interested in extending your study of this form you can find Yang Chengfu's detailed explanation of the whole form in *The Essence and Application of Taijiquan* translated by Louis Swain (2005)

6 GROUNDING AND SETTLING

The following static Chi Gung exercise is a commonly practised technique that can be utilised for several reasons:

i)   At the end of a session of moving meditation practice to help develop a basis for static calm-abiding meditation. For example, it can be substituted for the final posture of the 18 Postures Tai Chi-Chi Gung form.

ii) As a grounding and settling visualisation mechanism to relieve tension that often result from daily interactions, or to help discard the "infection" of negative emotions. With regard to the latter, it is particularly useful for individuals, e.g., medics, counsellors, carers, etc., who are exposed to people in emotionally negative states and environments.

iii) Simply to relax and tone things down at the end of the day.

iv) In Chi Gung circles, this is a method for ensuring correct balance of energy within certain vessels, which requires instruction from a Chi Gung master (for more detail see Liang & Wu, 1993 or Yang, 2014). However, one does not need to understand this method in order to gain benefit. The practice described below is appropriate for most individuals.

The Energy Shower

In this technique one uses the movements of the arms to assist the "mindful" visualisation of leading energy (Chi) throughout the body. It is worth mentioning, particularly to the sceptic, that for the purpose of this exercise and to achieve its effects, it matters not weather you believe in being able to connect with the energy of the environment or being able to lead it through the body and remove stagnant energy, etc. What matters is that you let go of your scepticism for a short while and just relax and give way to the visualisation for it to have its grounding and settling effects. Otherwise, don't bother; just keep taking the tablets Doctor! 😊

Outline of the Method

If one has mobility issues or when weak or tired, this exercise can usefully be performed sitting.

The following explanation summarises the simple hand movements which emphasise direction of energy flow. The physical movement along with the visualisation is conducive to mental grounding. The outline is followed by an explanation of a helpful visualisation process.

1. Stand with your feet shoulder-width apart and relax your arms and palms naturally at your sides. Unlock your knees slightly. Keep your baihui, huiyin and yongquan all in line (see Standing Posture 1).

2. Relax your visual attention slightly by lowering the gaze. Take one or two cleansing breaths to relax your mind and body and then breathe naturally until your mind is calm and your breathing is steady (see Appendix 5).

3. When relaxed and gently focused, raise both palms in a smooth arc over your head and turn the palms down.

4. Gently and slowly press the palms downward in front of your body until they are at your side. Repeat the movement.

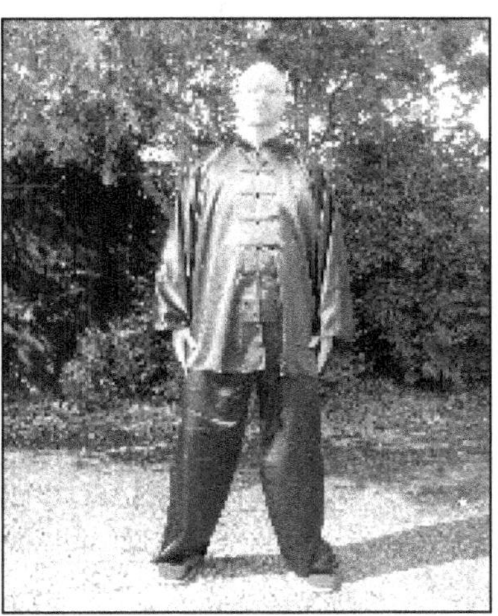
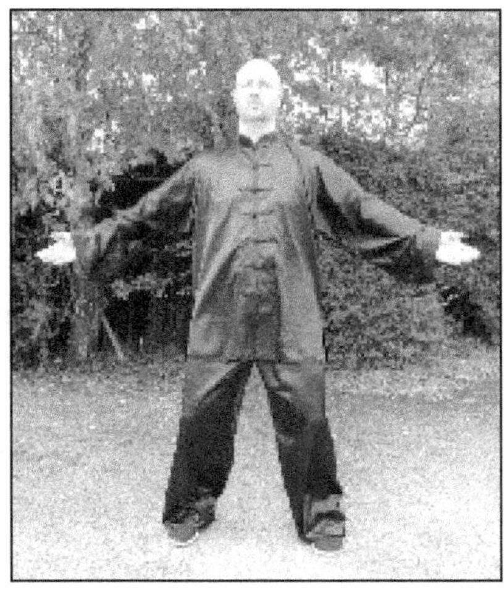

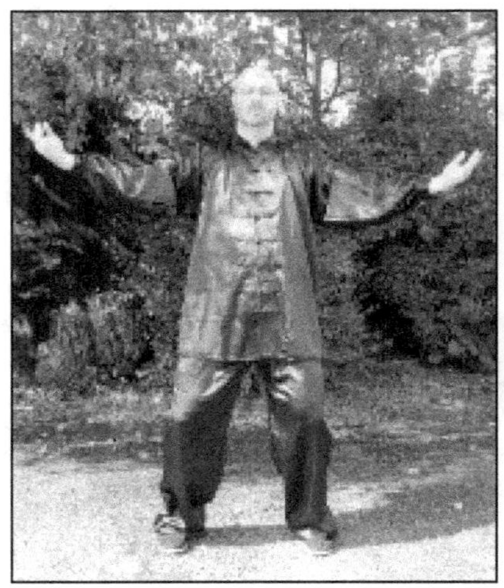 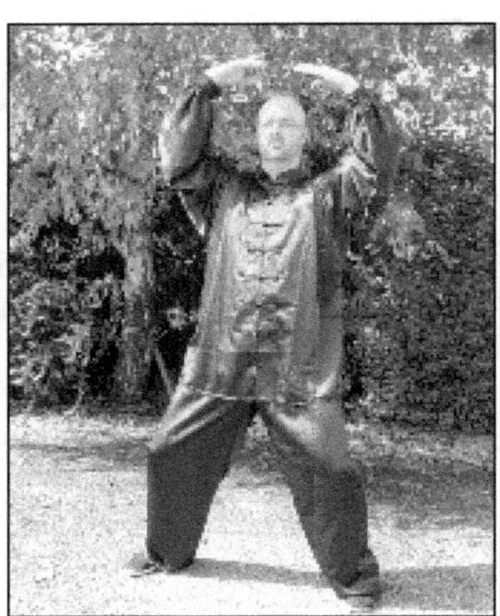

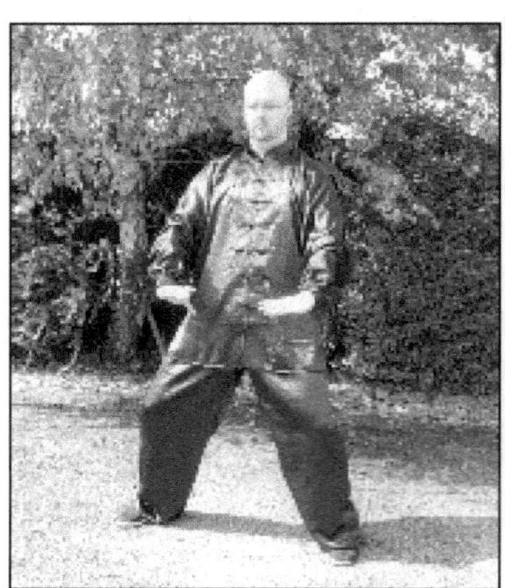 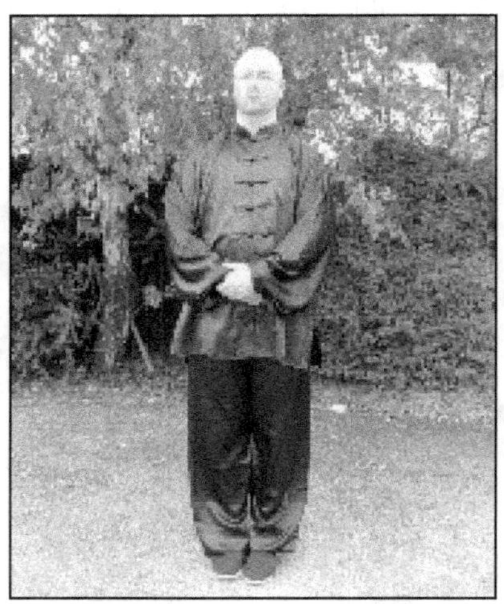

When you become more confident in yourself and with the technique, it is useful to practise in an open space beneath a large, healthy tree. Why not give it a try and see how it feels!!

Although I talk about this in appendix 8. I should emphasise here the vital need to be in touch with nature, particularly in the form of fresh air and sunlight. Any medical, scientific or government advice to the contrary must be flawed to say the least

Visualisation

Following a brief period of relaxation meditation in Basic Standing Posture 1 or 3, sweep the palms out with a confident and open countenance. Be very open and relaxed and as you slowly lift your palms visualise that you are connecting with and gathering the energy of the surrounding environment i.e., the earth, the air, and the trees, etc.

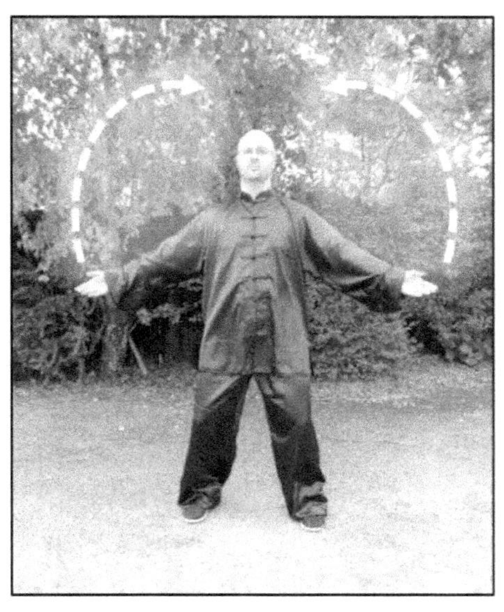

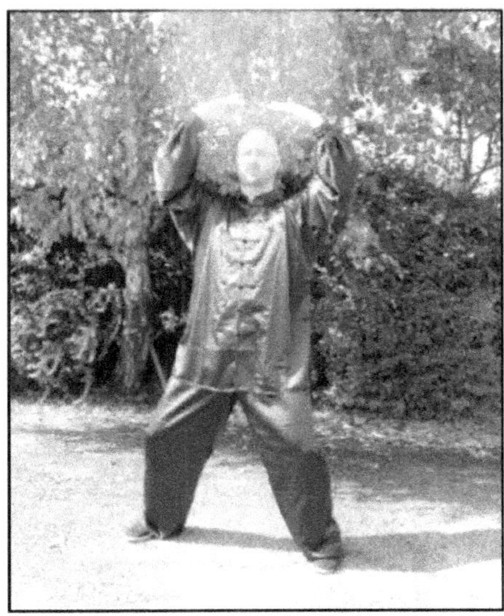

As your hands arrive above your head, visualise them breaking through the clouds where the radiant energy of the Sun (and the universe) is accessible. Now, the energy you have gathered in your palms, fuses with the energy of the Sun into a radiant, ethereal ball of white or golden light (whichever you prefer). The energy ball you have gathered in your palms connects with and leads, from above the palms, the radiant energy of the Sun.

As you slowly and gently press down the palms in front of your body you should try to gently visualise the ball of energy dissolving any tension or negativity in every part of your body. Begin at the scalp, then the brain/thoughts, the forehead, the eyebrows and eyes, ears, cheeks, lips, tongue chin, neck, shoulders, etc. Continue the visualisation, moving down through all areas of the torso, i.e., skin, muscles, bones, and organs.

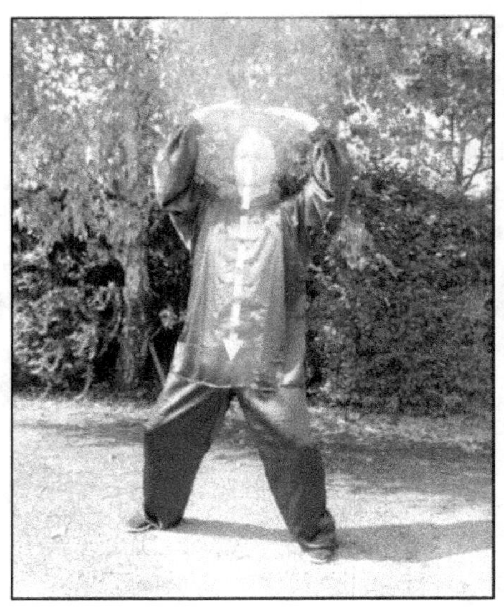

When the palms reach the hips, maintain a slight downward pressure as you continue the visualisation of tension /negativity being dissolved and displaced by the pure, "light" energy of the universe. Complete the visualisation down through the groin, backside and perineum, thighs, and legs, all the way to your feet. As you perform the visualisation, you may have the feeling of (or if not, at least visualise) the areas of your body above the palms becoming much clearer and lighter.

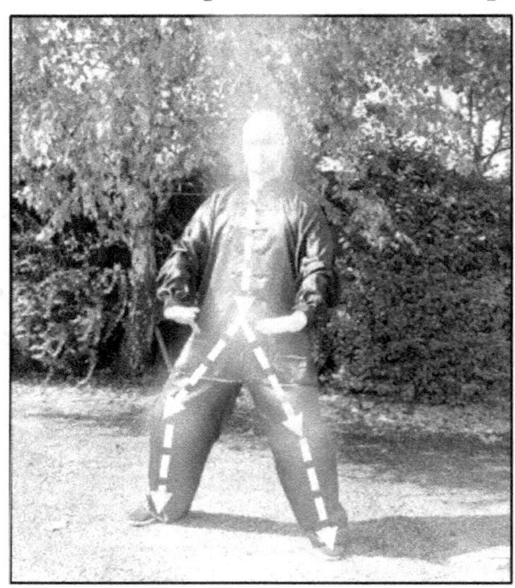

To complete the flow of energy and to ensure grounding and removal of negativity, the dissolved, displaced negative energy moves out through a visualised opening on the soles of the feet (*yongquan*), one metre into the earth where it is dissipated and neutralised in the vastness.

In short, as you do this, you visualise that the pure healing energy of the universe is filling all parts of your body and displacing tension and negativity or what we in Chi Gung might term energy stagnation. The visualisation of an energy ball in your palms is to dissolve and free up tension and negativity for subsequent displacement and replacement by the energy you are leading. Therefore, your palms should be moving continuously slightly in front of the main visualisation, "leading" the main energy visualisation behind them, not "pushing" it.

After completing one, two or three cycles, raise your heels off the floor lowering them gently or with a slight drop of the heels. This will help to relieve tension/pain in the feet that results from prolonged standing and will provide a gentle vibration throughout your body - a gentle shake to fully settle and relax things. At this point you might wish to stand peacefully with you palms facing each other in front of the dantien and place your attention between the palms to notice the concentration of Chi, which you might wish to use for the following massage.

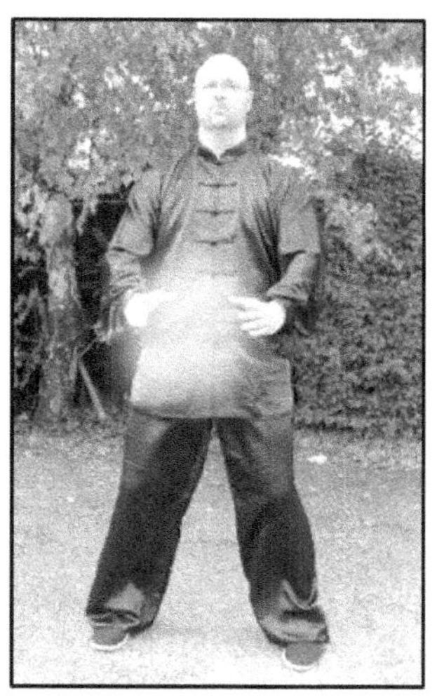

To close the form, breathe-in as you place your palms on the dantien, drawing your attention to that area at the same time. Finally, allow your breath to return to a natural rate and depth remaining in a relaxed, meditative state.

Alternatively, you can just pay gentle attention to your breath moving in and out. If you wish, you can finish at this point. Optionally and to greater effect, you can complete the exercises with a simple massage technique as follows.

Chi Gung Massage (Chi Wash)

"In the past, people practised the Tao, the Way of Life... Thus, they formulated practices such as... massaging... to promote energy flow..."
                          The Yellow Emperor's Classic of Medicine

The following describes a simplified adaptation of a more detailed method which requires guidance from a qualified teacher. However, for our purpose of general physical and mental health, the method provides a relaxing and gentle effleurage with its associated benefits. By way of completion of the above Chi Gung forms as part of a daily routine, this Chi Gung massage puts the finishing touches to the smooth and regulated flow of Chi elicited from practising the exercises. The gentle massage finally "smooths things out" and encourages the generation of "Guardian Chi", the surface emanation of Chi that helps to resist pathogenic influences. Or, if you are just into the materialist thing, it provides a soothing massage and completes nicely the relaxation-meditation of the previously practised Tai Chi and/or Chi Gung so that you can *"influence the pace of the daily rhythm in what we do, how we talk and think"*

The previous whole set of exercises, followed by massage, might be likened to building a fire in a grate or furnace, first you must clean the furnace and make sure there are no blocked grates or vents and pipes. Then you must light the fire using the energy containing materials you have, i.e., you give a boost of air to get the heat going and circulating around the room. However, once the fire is well lit, if you allow it to continue to burn in an uncontrolled manner, the temperature of your room would become too high and you will soon use up your energy source, so now you need to dampen it to a warm 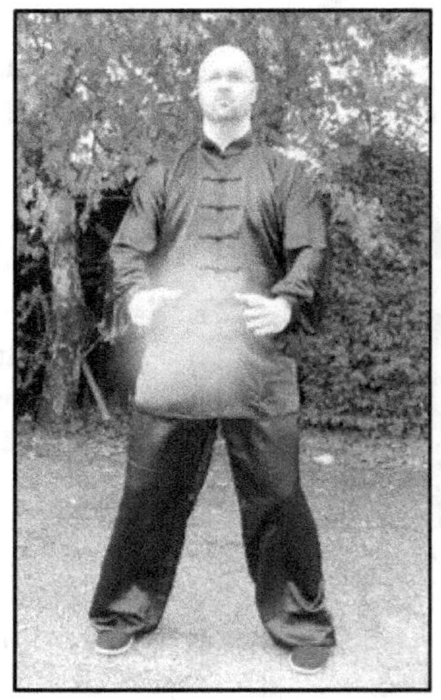 glow so that the energy release becomes steadily radiant and provides appropriate warmth. By doing this, the energy use is more efficient and effective over a longer period. But of course, you finally make sure that there are no bits and pieces around the fire that can inhibit the circulation of warmth in certain areas. Similar to this analogy, by practising the exercises, etc., we build our own internal fire and get the heat (Chi and fluids) circulating efficiently and effectively. Just to be sure that we clear any residual stagnation that might inhibit the optimal flow of energy (fluids and Chi), we use massage. By regular use of the exercises, along with the following massage technique we can help fend off disease caused by excess or deficient energy flow and furthermore, become more protected against the excesses of environmental wind, damp and cold.

So then, to finally clear the room and allow effective circulation of heat, so to speak, following the energy shower, stand in Basic Posture 1 or 2 with the Tai Chi palms facing each other. Keep your attention between the palms for a suitable period. You may or may not begin to get the feeling of some energy building up between the palms; if not, just visualise it. Now you can begin the Chi Gung Massage.

Separate the palms and place them flat on the chest, then you will slowly brush them over the neck, face, and scalp and down the back of the neck. The level of pressure used in the massage is up to the individual, but is should be quite light and soothing. Take care not to press hard on the sides of the neck. Throughout the massage, avoid any injured or inflamed areas, you can simply remove contact from those areas but still pass over them.

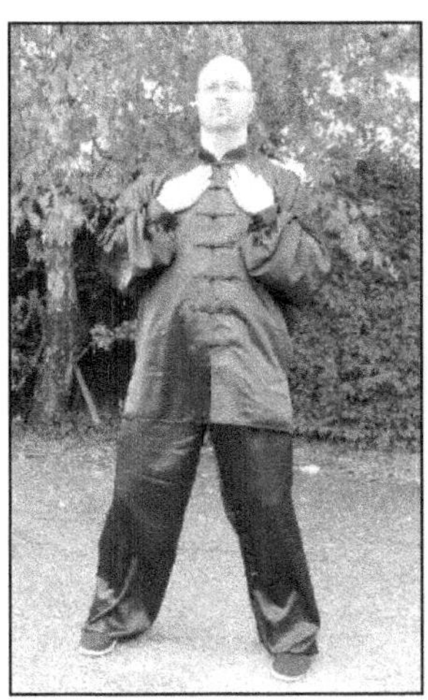
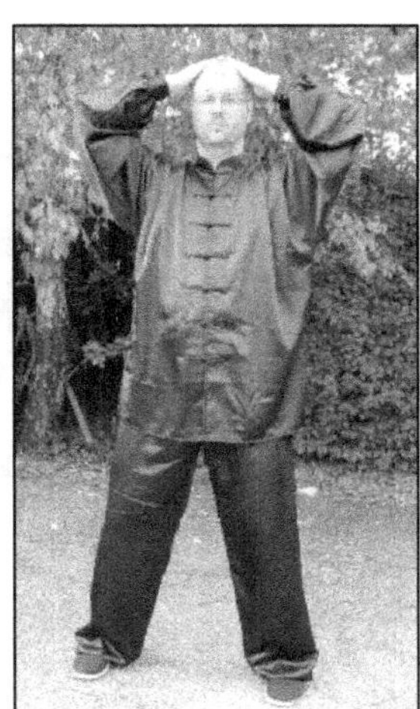
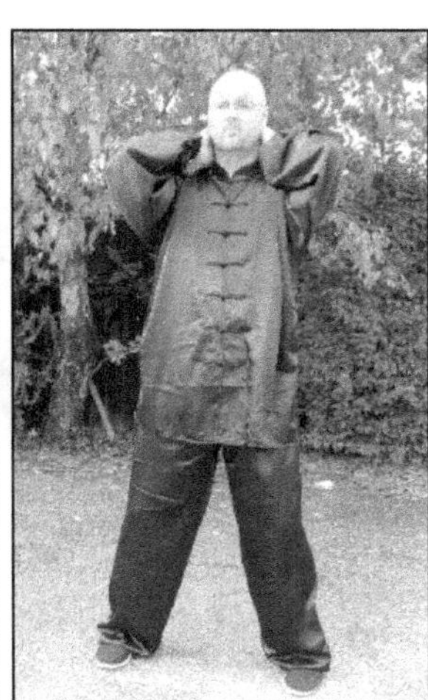

Now draw the palms over the neck and shoulders back down onto the chest. Keeping contact with the body, take the palms under the armpits and onto the back as high as you can above the kidneys and down the lumbar area with thumbs over the flanks. Now draw them over the sacrum and backside and down the back of the thighs and legs, with the thumbs brushing over the outer aspects of the legs.

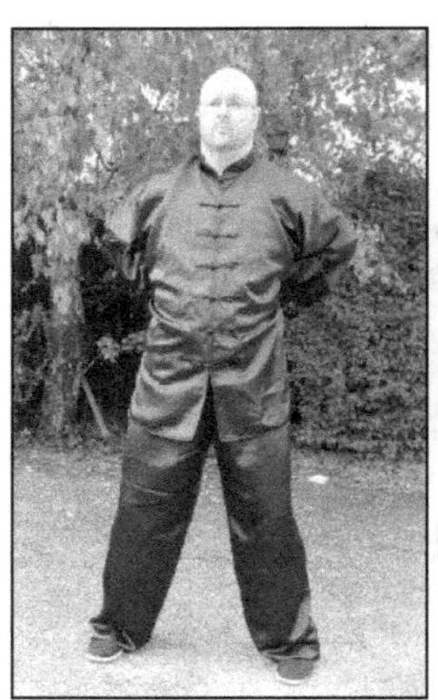
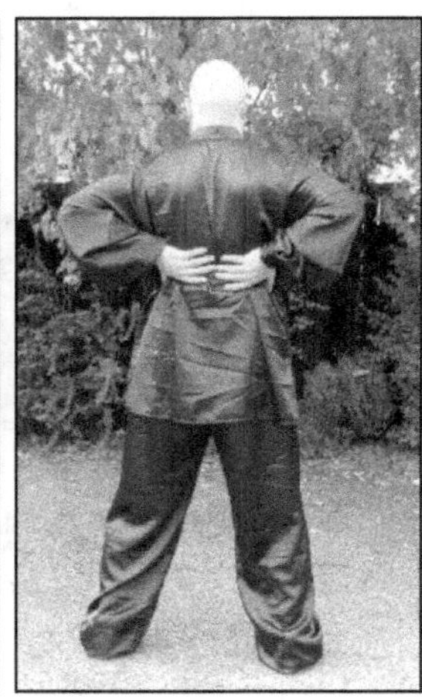
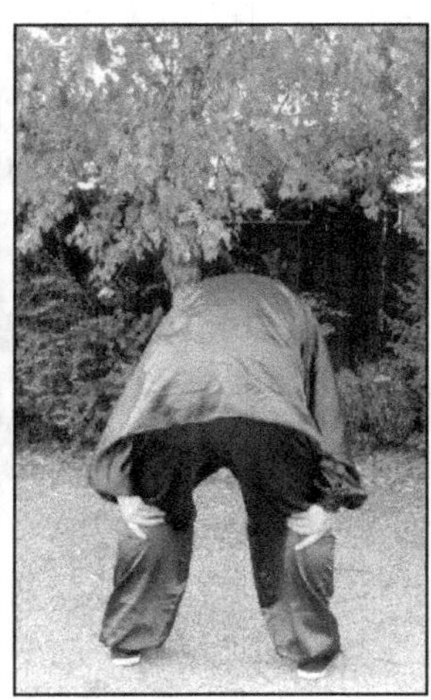

Continue by brushing over the ankles and dorsal aspect of the feet then up the legs and thighs into the groin up the abdomen and over the chest. Repeat the cycle a few times.

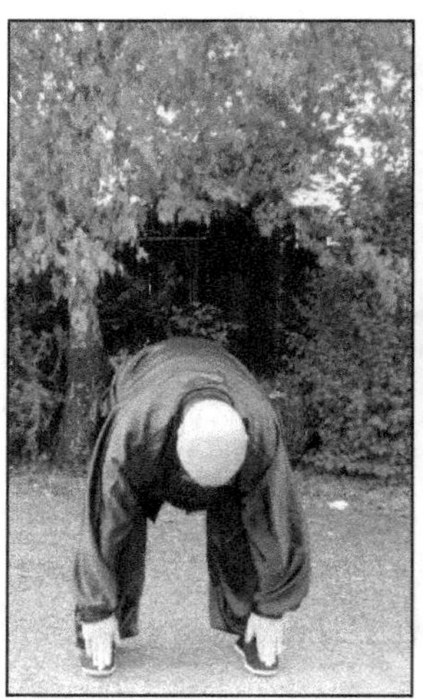
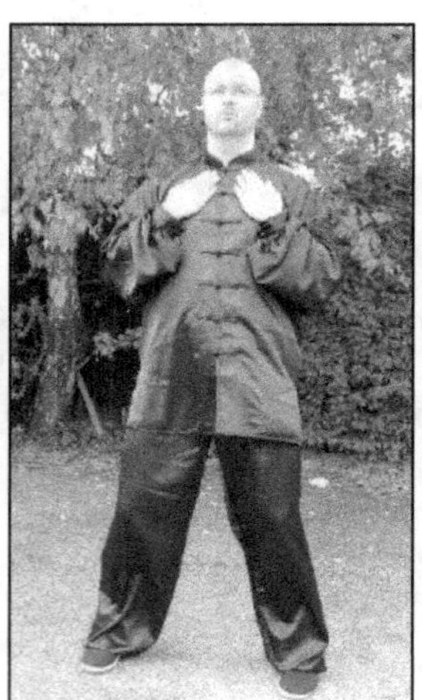
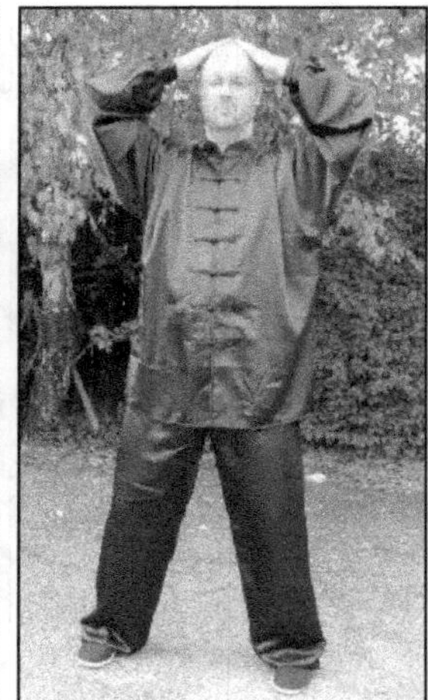

Finish the massage by brushing over the face and scalp once more, back down the neck and press the palms down to face each other once more at the dantien level, then close the energy ball into the dantien.

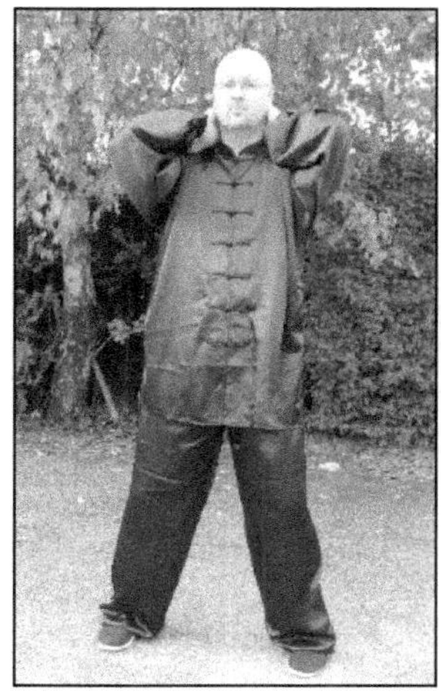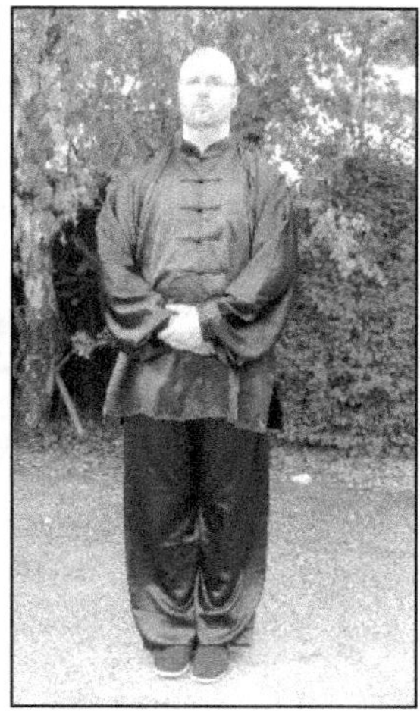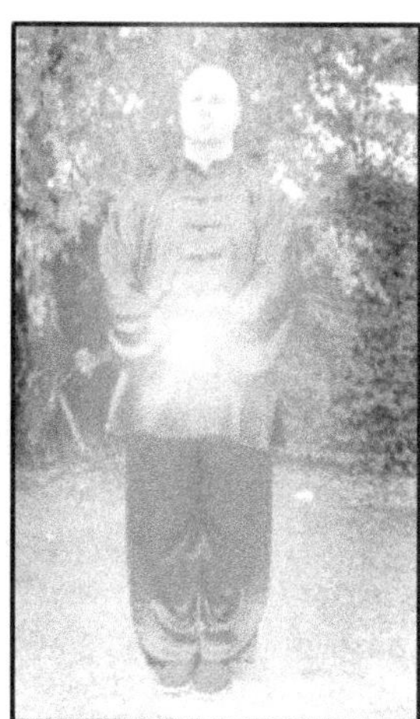

As you close the palms in, draw your attention to the dantien. Now consider that firstly, you generally loosened any tension and areas of stagnation, warming-up ready for the Chi Gung. Then, the slow meditative action of the Chi Gung removed blockages and lesions and opened up areas of stagnation, mobilising Chi and fluids more effectively. Following on, you settled everything and removed any remaining stagnation and negativity and smoothed out the flow of energy.

Finally, meditate that the energy at the dantien is now functioning optimally, like a fire burning efficiently. Consequently, the energy source gently radiates and thus circulates freely, yet efficiently, and begins to emit from all your body pores with a gentle glow i.e., "Guardian Chi". Stand or sit meditating on your gently radiant form for a comfortable length of time.

****

So, there it is, "Tai Chi for YOU". Remember, for it to have some effect, YOU must do it. Happy Tai Chi!!

APPENDIX 1. SUN STYLE TAI CHI - BACKGROUND

Sun Style Tai Chi was developed by the famous scholar and martial artist known as Sun Lutang. Master Sun was born in Hebei and was named Sun Fuquan. He studied Xing Yi Chuan with Li Kuiyuan and Guo Yunshen, and Baguazhang with Cheng Tinghua (who gave him the name Lutang). Relatively later in life, Sun learned Wu (Hao) style Tai Chi Chuan from Hao Wei-chen.

Master Sun's unique system is clearly based on Hao style but heavily influenced by Xing Yi and Bagua. It has a characteristic follow-through step-up, which is associated with the follow-through often found in martial application of other systems but not in the forms themselves. This characteristic step makes it slightly easier to perform for more senior folk, without losing any of the effectiveness of the weight bearing postures.

Much of this background information was kindly provided to me by my teacher Bob Melia.

Many Fylde Tai Chi Association members were fortunate to have studied Sun style directly from Bob Melia and consequently received authentic teachings in an unbroken lineage. The section of the form in Chapter 5 was adapted by me for beginners and to aid learning of official training forms and long form. For more information about Sifu Bob Melia and Sun Style or to arrange seminars in this and other systems see Direct Essence Boxing International currently at http://www.warriorarts.net/.

Sun Lutang's own writings on Sun style can be found in Tim Cartmell's 2003 translation of *A Study of Tajiquan*.

APPENDIX 2. YANG STYLE TAI CHI – BACKGROUND

Yang Tai Chi is, arguably, the most popular form of Tai Chi practised in the West. Its slow graceful movements have contributed to the popular esoteric image of Tai Chi in the consciousness of people searching for profound method of mental peace or simply an exercise programme which contributes to a healthy mind and body. Its precursor, the also popular Chen family style, is graceful but, arguably, a little more strenuous tending towards Wushu and often, but not necessarily, lends itself to the younger more athletic practitioner. Yang style developed from Chen Tai Chi. As with all Gung Fu systems their origins are not fully clear, but it is known that Yang Luchan (1700-1872) studied Chen and from that developed the characteristic Yang family style. In the lineage, Yang Luchan's grandson Yang Chengfu (1883-1936) was perhaps the most important teacher in the popularisation of Yang family style leading to its current popularity.

Perhaps most notably, Yang style's popularity became dominant in the West because of the efforts of Yang Lu Chan's student Cheng Manching and his American student Robert Smith. The wonderful teacher who first introduced me and other fortunate students to the internal arts in the early 1970's and in particular Yang Tai Chi was Miss Rose Li.

Yang Chengfu's own writings on Yang style can be found in Louis Swain's 2005 translation of *Essence and Applications of Taijiquan*.

APPENDIX 3. ZHAN ZHUANG – OVERVIEW

Zhan Zhuang is a form of standing Chi Gung, one might say "standing meditation". The martial artist, in addition to having clarity of mind, must develop internal and external strength and power and so several Chi Gung methods were developed for this purpose. As with all Chinese martial arts, particularly the internal arts, the methods have been shown to be beneficial for mental and physical health and wellbeing. Zhan Zhuang is a Chi Gung method commonly utilised in *Xing Yi* and *Yi Chuan* for the above purpose but is now used for general fitness purposes, physical resistance to illness and medical recovery.

Although only one position is shown in our text there are several hand positions and a few stances utilised, but all have the characteristic of a strong foundation, confident strength, and stillness. The basic stance utilises the correct postural alignment as outlined in the text with regard to *mabu*. Here, I shall elaborate slightly. In general, try to ensure a parallel position of all relevant points, i.e., they are in line. For example, in addition to the points mentioned earlier in the text, the feet should be parallel and in line with the crease at the femoral angle (*Kua*). The knees should be in line with the feet and should not flex beyond the toes. The mind and body should be relaxed but there is a focus on relaxation of the chest and abdomen and heaviness of the legs.

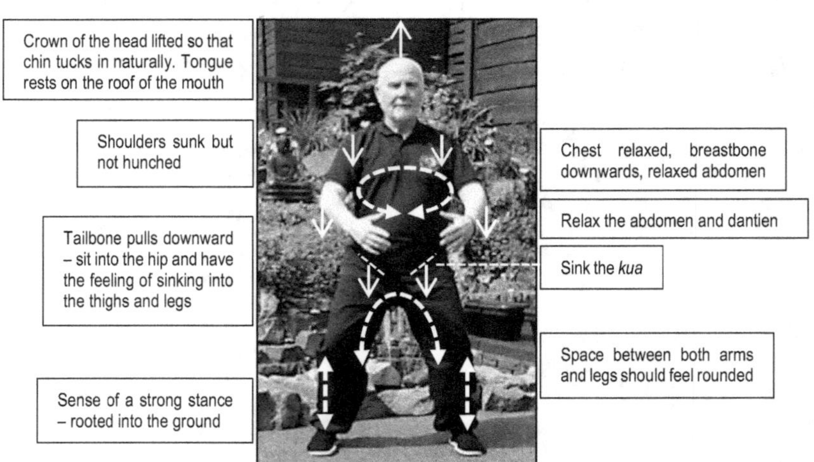

For a detailed introduction to Zhan Zhuang see *The Way of Energy*, Lam Kam Chuen (1991)

APPENDIX 4. TOWARDS A HEALTHY ROUTINE

Before embarking upon practise, you should study all the points below:

• If you are suffering from an acute illness you should refrain from practise and consult your doctor or other appropriate health-care provider.

• If you are suffering from a chronic complaint and unsure how Chi Gung might affect it, consult your doctor or other appropriate health-care provider.

• Try not to smoke. Medical advice suggests that smoking can cause lung and associated disease. As effective natural breathing is of primary importance in the practise of Chi Gung, it is wise to resist the temptation to smoke, particularly prior to practise, as nicotine can cause unwanted stimulation of breathing rate and restriction of airways. Although, smoking is known to have a relaxing effect, it is also known to stimulate release of the very stress chemicals that are the result of, and which exacerbate, the *"frantic pace of modern life"*

• Do not practise on a full or empty stomach. On the one hand, the energy of your body should not be distracted by dealing with digesting a large meal while you are exercising but on the other hand, your mind should not be distracted by hunger and thirst.

• Although we use Tai Chi and Chi Gung to relax and reduce anxiety and stress, it is best not to practise immediately on becoming upset or anxious as it will be of little benefit and can be harmful. Stabilise your mood first by doing some easy exercises. The stretching and mobilising exercises in chapter 2 & 3 or just the arm swinging is useful for this. It will at least distract you from your problems, help defuse your strong emotions and allow you to relax a little.

• Beginners should not practise too excessively or intensely at first. Regular, small workouts are much more effective than sudden bursts. This will help to develop a regular habit and gradually, gradually, you can increase the repetition and extent of the postures.

• Wear loose, comfortable clothing and light but supportive footwear. Tai Chi can be practised barefoot, but this should not be on a cold floor. If practising barefooted outdoors, you should do so on a sandy beach or soft grass in warm weather: not on a cold hard floor!

• Try to practise in a place conducive to relaxation, i.e., pleasant, peaceful surroundings. A nice quiet garden or other natural environment. These days, folk tend not to bother you when practicing in a park or on a beach.

• Avoid practising outdoors in bad weather, particularly electrical storms, or windy conditions. Chi is adversely affected by such conditions - especially if you get struck by lightning!

• If you cannot practice outdoors and must practise indoors, avoid distractions, and keep any environment in which you practise well ventilated. DO NOT wear a mask when practising. If it is that you must or feel you must wear a mask, FORGET IT, and do something else!

• Before practise, warm up and loosen joints and muscles. Although the movements of Tai Chi and Chi Gung are gentle, some are strenuous and require a degree of control, stretching and twisting. Warming up will help prepare for this and help prevent injury. The exercises in chapter 2 & 3 are useful for this purpose.

• Practise only within your own physical limitations. We all have different physical abilities and limitations, do not try to stretch beyond your capabilities or push yourself too far. This is against the principles of "no extremes" and natural harmonious movement. If you feel unwell or unusually tired during practise, take a break!

• At first, once you have learned some Tai Chi and Chi Gung, it can start to feel repetitive and boring, and our busy little minds often want to find something more interesting to do. However, if you persevere, this distraction will eventually be overcome.

• Try not to become apathetic towards your practise. The simple and repetitive exercises of Chi Gung belie their effectiveness. Chi

Gung is an ongoing process of development, and we derive benefit each time we practise correctly - at any level.

• There is only one way to benefit from Chi Gung and that is to practise what you have learned. Avoid becoming obsessive but try to build a regular routine. It is quite difficult at first to recall the full sequences so practise the postures you know until they become easy to remember, then you be able to concentrate on what you have forgotten or on new postures.

• To achieve improved health through Chi Gung you must be willing to spend some time on a regular basis, each day if possible. It might seem like a task at first but in the end, you will gain more than the initial effort because of improved health and a calmer mind.

In Brief

Pay attention to the above but in general begin by gently loosening and stretching the joints and muscles and mobilising fluids. Especially, you should never practise Chi Gung when highly agitated, so it is best to do some warm-up Chi Gung and help to use up the stress chemicals. Before practising it is helpful to relax into the basic posture, cleanse the breath and calm the mind and body (See chapter 2 and appendix 5) and give yourself some space to enable you to focus on the main Chi Gung form

APPENDIX 5. CORRECT NATURAL BREATHING

One should keep in mind three key elements to work with in Chi Gung practise for health: body, breath, and mind. Correct graded practise in Chi Gung concentrates firstly on adjusting the body, discussed in the main text (this includes relaxation, flexibility, and mobility); then regulated (natural) breathing; then focussing the mind (attentive and present - currently identified as mindfulness). Always keep in mind, they are not separate, and working on one affects the others. As the classics state, *"When the shape* (referring to body and its functions) *is wrong, then Chi* (energy flow and manifestation) *will not be smooth, when Chi is not smooth the mind will not be peaceful,"* and *"mind and breath are mutually dependent"* (See books by Yang Jwing Ming). The main text was focussed on the body, specifically movement, but as Yang implies focusing on the body alone is incomplete.

Mind and Breath Affect Each Other
Although alluded to earlier, it is perhaps worthwhile at this point to elaborate a little. According to Taoist alchemy, the breath acts like a bellows to power the transformation and movement of subtle energies, which can further be assisted by movements of the body, such as those of Dao yin, Chi Gung and Tai Chi (See Da Liu, 1974). Notwithstanding this spiritual aspect, for everyday folk, such natural, deep breathing methods when combined with specific movement and postures, is sufficient to contribute to good mental and physical health. So, whether for spiritual or health purposes, relaxed, effective, natural breathing is central.

Undoubtedly, even within the Western physiological model, there is a strong connection between mind and breath: our thought states are reflected in our breath patterns. For example, pain in the body and emotional states are often accompanied by marked changes in breathing rate. When we are in a confrontational or stressed state we may breathe more rapidly and tend to exhale more strongly than we inhale. In short, the lungs react to our mental state and give rise to the outward expression of everything we feel, e.g., when we speak, laugh or cry. This mind and breath connection can be seen from a Western scientific point of view in Figure 5 below. The brain receives information from the senses and interprets that information as a threat or otherwise, this then causes stimulation of the neural pathways to the muscles of respiration and the airways, which in turn causes the airways to dilate (or in some abnormal cases, constrict) and the breathing rate to increase.

The simplified diagram below suggests how our mind can affect the way we breathe. Conversely, empirical, and anecdotal evidence shows that the way we breathe can affect our mind. This can be seen from the example mentioned earlier, when we are nervous or agitated, we often take a deep breath followed by a full, slow, exhalation, which seems to help settle the nervous tension and thus, calm the mind (sometimes termed a "cleansing breath").

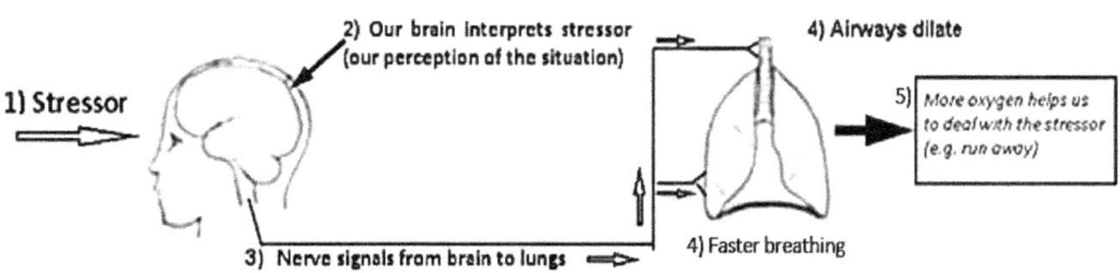

Figure 5. *Shows how the mind affects the breathing process 1) Visual perception of a stressor 2) The brain interprets the visual perception as exciting or dangerous 3) Nerve signals are transmitted from the brain to the lungs 4) Airways dilate and breathing rate increases 5) Dilation of airways and increased breathing rate increases the delivery and uptake of oxygen into the blood. Therefore, our perception of danger causes us to breathe faster and deeper. Conversely, when we feel safe and comfortable, our breathing slows down and becomes accordingly shallower.*

So then, if breath is not calm, the mind will not be calm and, according to Chi Gung theory, Chi will not flow smoothly. By calming our breathing, we can calm the mind. It is this mechanism which Chi Gung utilises to achieve a certain state of mental clarity, sometimes referred to as "mindfulness" the state when *Hsin* - the emotional or agitated mind, has settled and *Yi* - the wisdom mind, can start to become clearer. Therefore, we can say, the purpose of Chi Gung is to co-ordinate mind, body, and breath more effectively in order to improve and enhance the efficient use and flow of Chi.

Earlier, we gained some understanding of how to relax or "regulate" the breath. Although many of us must "re-learn" to breathe more optimally and effectively, it is important when practising Chi

Gung that the breath pattern should be natural and uncontrived. Through guidance and regular practise, our physical foundation becomes stronger and the movements of Chi Gung become smoother and more relaxed, the mind becomes calmer and the breath smoother and more even. Once this occurs, we can learn to co-ordinate our breathing more effectively by utilising "abdominal breathing" methods.

The theory of abdominal breathing and breath co-ordination in Chi Gung and Tai Chi is ostensibly simple. Commonly, a *yang* or outward physical action is accompanied by a *yang* breath or exhalation; a yin or withdrawing movement is accompanied by a yin breath or inhalation. (The opposite can sometimes apply depending on posture and purpose). However, practise is not so simple, those who attempt breath co-ordination too early may develop tension, gross or subtle, in the body and breathing, and consequently the mind. It is not uncommon for a beginner to be too controlling and to breathe too deeply, or even for the breath to become tight and shallow. Both types of inappropriate breathing can adversely affect the use and flow of Chi and, from the Western medical perspective, the chemical nature (pH) of body fluids. An abnormal fluctuation in pH can adversely affect the function and health of our cells and tissues with a consequent adverse effect on the way we feel and think (see Further Notes on Breathing below)

Like all Chi Gung methods, correctly regulated breathing should be developed in a gradual manner and certainly under the guidance of a competent teacher. Concerning relaxation and regulation of breath, it is best for the beginner to stand or sit for a short while in the correct posture and just allow the body to be naturally extended and open. In this comfortable posture, allow your mind and breath to calm. When one begins the exercise, it is best to not focus on any pattern but to just keep the breath relaxed and follow a natural breath.

How to develop natural breathing for Tai Chi and Chi Gung
Sit or stand as in Posture 1 or Posture 2. A useful position for the hands when cleansing and calming the breath is shown in Basic Standing Posture 3 & appendix 3, or simply rest them on the dantien.

1. Firstly, take a deeper than normal in-breath and breathe out through the nose or blow out through the mouth, whichever way feels most relaxing and settling. One, two or three times is enough to "cleanse" the breath. Try to use the diaphragm muscles followed by, but in unison with, the chest muscles, i.e., feel the abdomen expand followed by the chest. Do not force this, it should be quite comfortable (see Figure 6 below).

2. Initially, hold your gaze at a point that feels comfortable, e.g., slightly in front of your nose or ahead.

3. Gently breathe in and out through the nose*.

4. As you breathe in, visualise the breath moving in a gentle stream, filling your skull, brain, and your whole body. You can imagine the air in the form of a soothing white light if it is helpful. As this happens, imagine the air is having a soothing effect on all the agitation and tension in your mind and body. As you breathe in, it is helpful to think of the word *calm*.

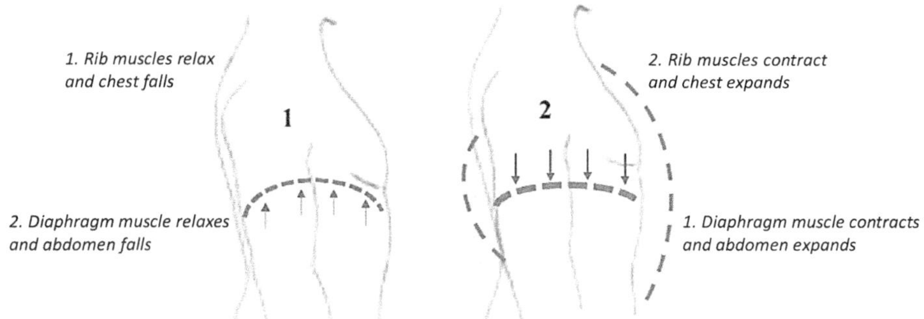

Figure 6. 1) *Exhaling – the rib muscles relax, and the diaphragm muscle relax causing an out-breath. 2) Inhaling - the diaphragm muscle contracts, and the rib muscles contract causing an out-breath. Effective diaphragmatic breathing ('abdominal breathing') is essential to regulation of Chi, the movement of fluids and effective oxygenation of tissues.*

5. Now, imagine that the soothing calming air or light has dissolved and soaked up all the mental and physical tension and agitation. As you breathe out through the nose*, visualise the breath or light transporting all the dissolved tension and agitation out of your mind and body leaving them feeling nice

and relaxed. As you breathe out, it is helpful to think of the word *relax*.

6. Do this a few times until your mind and body start to feel relaxed, and you are ready to focus on any postures. You can use this technique for longer periods to aid relaxation but if you spend too long before doing the warmups, you might become too relaxed and not want to do the exercise! This is a useful first step in learning to relax and regulate the breath for Tai Chi practice.

**It is best to breathe in and out through the nose but if you have difficulty breathing through the nose only, then it is fine to use the mouth as well.*

Further Notes on Breathing

The   nature of normal or abnormal breathing depends upon conditions and circumstances, e.g., activity or pathology, what is normal and abnormal is a complex discussion and best left to respiratory specialist, nurses, and physiotherapists, especially with regard to respiratory pathology.

For the general purposes of Tai Chi and Chi Gung, breathing should relate to the level of exercise but should never be rapid and shallow and, except for the increased requirements of oxygen and removal of carbon dioxide in active Wushu and martial application or any exercise, nor should it be rapid and deep. For the purposes of Tai Chi and Chi Gung for health one should always be mindful of the advice that *"mind and breath are mutually dependent"*. Consequently, if breath is calm and deep, mind will be calm and deep and vice-versa: thus, balance is essential.

Other than for specific yogic techniques, which have a more spiritual emphasis and should be for those committed to such a path and carried out under the guidance of a master, for our purposes we should generally aim for slower, deeper breathing without it being contrived or forced. This takes some degree of attention and practise at first before it becomes more natural. It is helpful to bear in mind the Tai Chi symbol with regard to the balanced approach to breathing.

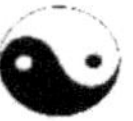

1. Normal Breathing

The diagram below represents the pattern of breathing in wave form. The in-breath appears to reach a peak and then changes to the out-breath. In fact, in healthy adult breathing, the in-breath FLOWS into the out-breath without stopping or suddenly changing, although this imperceptible flow is normally only perceived as a sudden change. Sudden, rasping change is indicative of pathology. Normal adult breathing rate is approximately 12-16 breaths per minute.

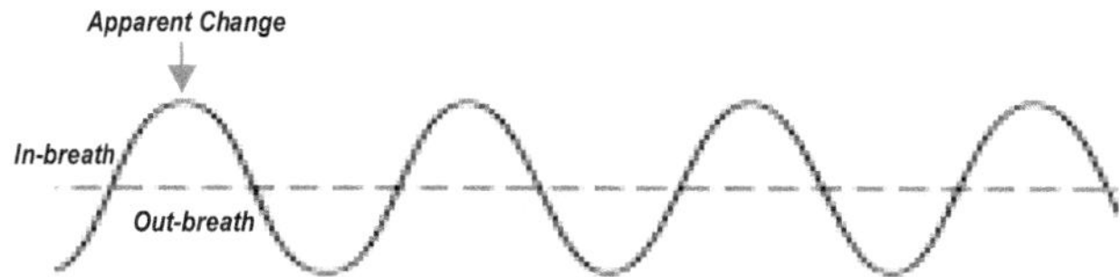

Under normal conditions the in-breath utilises the external rib muscles and diaphragm to breath in but the out-breath results from their relaxation (See figure 6).

2. Rapid Breathing

Rapid, deep breathing following active exercise requires a more rapid and forceful change from in-breath to out-breath. This type of breath in the absence of activity suggests *hyperventilation,* as in anxiety or certain medical conditions. This can affect pH of body fluids adversely and so, other than because of activity or excitement, it should be avoided or addressed.

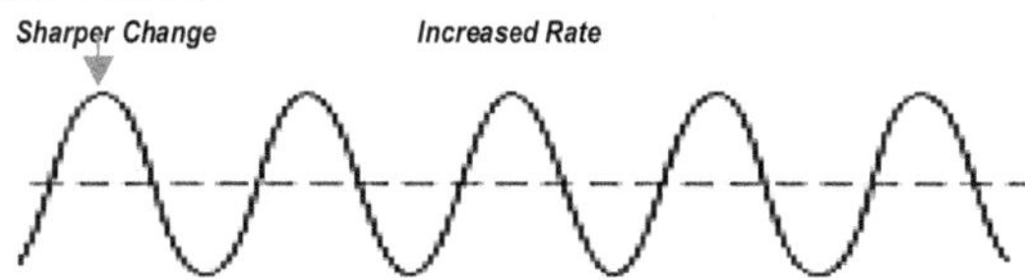

Rapid shallow breathing is indicative of a pathology e.g., COPD, pneumonia, pain, etc.

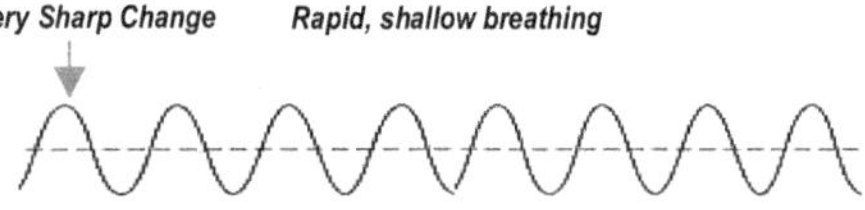

Rapid breathing requires the use of the internal muscles of the rib to force air out quickly. The natural flow from in to out is quicker and sharper. If this condition occurs in the absence of a normal reason such as exercise, it requires medical attention.

3.   Breathing Rate and Depth in Tai Chi and Chi Gung

I must re-emphasise that regulating the breath in Tai Chi requires direct tuition from a competent teacher so that it is *regulated* "naturally" and not controlled, contrived, or forced "unnaturally".

As I have indicated, under normal conditions, the rate and depth of breathing should be in keeping with the level of activity and prevailing conditions. A person in good health tends to adjust accordingly and naturally. However, in Tai Chi and Chi Gung we attempt to enhance nature or at least prevent or reverse the natural tendency for breathing to become less efficient with age or illness. Master Yang Jwing Ming pointed out quite starkly that as we age there is a tendency to move away from the optimal deep breathing mechanism of the healthy child, who tends to breath with the whole of the torso, to breathing with the chest, until, depending on the individual's state of health, the breathing becomes much higher in the chest and shallower with the potential for adverse health consequences. Beyond that the outlook is poor! Thus, in Chi Gung we encourage a *Return to Childhood Breathing* in order to promote life extension and health enhancement.

The process mentioned earlier and the use of effective diaphragmatic breathing, contribute greatly to enhanced natural breathing in Tai Chi and Chi Gung but now, having a little more insight into breathing patterns, we might see how we can contribute further to natural slow, deeper breathing that can be coordinated with the movements of Tai Chi and Chi Gung, thus enhancing the flow of Chi without causing adverse effects of forced, deep breathing.

To breath more slowly, especially to coordinate the breath with the postures, in-breath and out-breath are extended (not necessarily deeper, although this will naturally occur in the breathing cycles). Importantly, the change from in to out and out to in is naturally prolonged so that you might feel there is a gap. But this is not the case, it is simply that the change from in-breath (yin) to out-breath (yang) is so smooth and refined that it seems imperceptible.

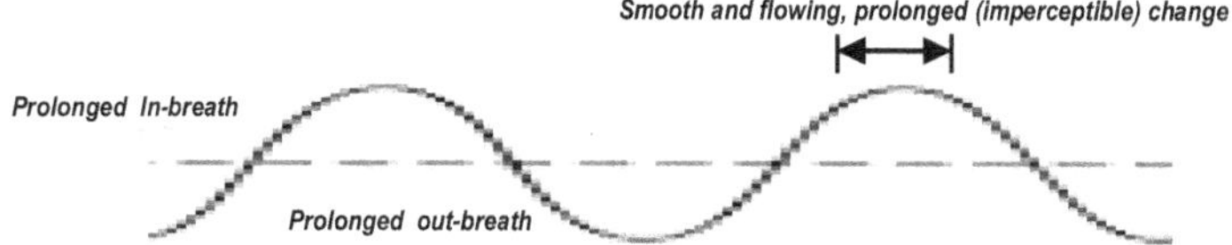

So now we can see the slow, flowing yin and yang relationship of the slow, flowing in-breath and out-breath.

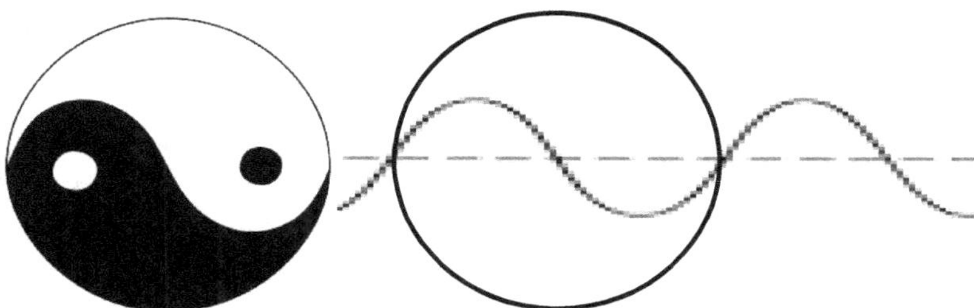

This then is the nature of the slower, deeper breathing of Tai Chi and Chi Gung which results from the use of the whole of the torso in *Return to Childhood Breathing* method. This, along with Tai Chi's slowing down exercises, in the words of Nyanaponika Mahathera, is *"…helpful in reducing mental and physical tension…"* and can *"…influence the pace of the daily rhythm in what we do, how we talk and think"*

When trained in this method by a competent teacher, one can begin to coordinate the slower but optimal, natural breath with the movements of Tai Chi and Chi Gung to optimum effect, which is primarily to enhance the flow of Chi or life-force in the vessels and organs, which in turn will beneficially affect our anatomy and physiology. In any event, with or without coordinated breathing, the benefits of Tai Chi and Chi Gung will become apparent, provided one applies oneself to regular practise, employs natural relaxed breathing, and addresses correct posture and mindfulness.

APPENDIX 6. MINDFULNESS IN MOVEMENT

Any attempt to engender optimum health and ameliorate or cure disease, should acknowledge the vital relationship between mind and body and the energies underlying and facilitating their interdependent activities: simply, how the state of one affects the state of the other. Importantly, within Chi Gung theory, it seems that within and for a harmonious interplay of all elements, the state of mind is of prime importance if optimum health is to be achieved in any given circumstances. *The Yellow Emperor's Classic of Internal Medicine* states:

"When internal energies are able to circulate smoothly and freely, and the energy of the mind is not scattered, but focused and concentrated, illness and disease can be avoided" (Maoshing, Ni. 1995).

Also recall, *"When the shape is wrong, then Chi will not be smooth, when Chi is not smooth the mind will not be peaceful,"* and *"mind and breath are mutually dependent"* (Yang Jwing Ming, 1998).

As a matter of fact, in most "holistic" systems of health, mind plays a key role. Although the concept of "mind" can be profound and complex and so beyond the scope of this book, understanding the importance of a calm and clear mind (in the everyday sense of the word) in Tai Chi and Chi Gung is essential to both physical and mental health. The methods clearly employ positive mental intention; because of this, such exercises have been termed "moving meditation" or "meditation in action". The meditative aspect of the movements engenders clarity of mind, calms the emotions and consequently, invigorates the spirit. It is this aspect of Chi Gung that helps to develop a healthy, co-ordinated mind and body that *"is not scattered, but focused and concentrated"* and thus, better able to deal with the pathogenic stressors which individuals may encounter in their daily lives.

In Chi Gung theory, there is often no distinction between physical and mental disease, as a physical dysfunction can cause mental disharmony; conversely, mental disharmony can cause physical problems (see Appendix 8). The movements of Chi Gung, when performed with meditative intention, enable the practitioner to relax the mind and body at deeper levels, assisting in the removal of more chronic or subtle tensions that may build up as a result of the increasing stress and pace of modern life.

So then, the dynamic movements of Tai Chi and Chi Gung, while providing a useful physical exercise, also provide an emphasis for mental focus that can help develop a calm and peaceful mind but in turn, a calm and peaceful mind further enhances the health effects of the movements by directing *"internal energies… to circulate smoothly and freely."* Master John Farrell points out, *"…In one sense, the character of the movement is less important, any 'complete' set of movements will suffice provided that they are generated from a strong root, performed correctly and with mindfulness".* Suggesting that whatever form one adopts, providing it is performed in the prescribed manner and one avoids distraction and applies attention and focus, benefits will ensue.

From a relatively new, evidence-based, medical point of view, any form of meditation done correctly, to a greater or lesser degree, causes our neurophysiology (nervous system) and consequently our somatic physiology (body) to switch from a state of alertness and action (mental and physical responses to living, which can be healthy if moderate, short term and resolved but pathological if excessive, prolonged and unresolved – a frequent effect of the *"frantic pace, modern life"*) to a more "restful" state, which has a beneficial effect on mind and body and consequently, emotions. This is perhaps one of the reasons why the current "mindfulness movement" along with some of the old standbys such as Yoga and our own Tai Chi and Chi Gung have risen in popularity.

It is worth mentioning at this point that there are limitations with regard to the psychological/emotional health effects of such methods as much of the stress and anxiety we experience arises from our disordered or incorrect view of life and no amount of mindfulness meditation, Tai Chi or Yoga exercise alone will address these issues fully. Perhaps the most profound method of developing mindfulness, which is beyond the scope of the modern (secular) mindfulness movement and Tai Chi, etc. (which undoubtedly have their uses in healthcare) is what is known in Buddhist circles as "calm-abiding meditation" or *shamatha*. The ultimate purpose of such meditation is to address the primary or root causes of the emotional states, which happen to manifest in stress, anxiety, and unhappiness. How can this be and what is it that is different from secular mindfulness, etc.? As the meditation master Lama Jampa Thaye (2018) explains, *"The actual qualities of gentleness, stillness, calmness and stability that arise through meditation are not possible on the basis of a disordered indulgent life, so our behaviour also needs to change."* Although this is an issue beyond the remit and scope of this book, nevertheless, it is worth mentioning for those seeking to find a more lasting peace of mind beyond mundane physical and mental health.

This important limitation notwithstanding, there are undeniable, and quite profound, emotional, and physical health benefits to the practise of Tai Chi and Chi Gung. In this author's experience, with regard to developing mindfulness, Tai Chi can be helpful for those of us who are easily distracted and find it difficult to remain still for long periods. By being a slowing down "activity" and "distraction-like" object of focus, Tai Chi can at least begin to cultivate a physical and mental attitude that might eventually be conducive to a more equanimous approach to life. As the monk Nynaponika Mahathera advised,

"...it is imperative that, in our free time, we try consciously to pause and slow down... slowing down is helpful in reducing mental and physical tension... Beyond the immediate effects of an exercise session, slowing down exercises influence the pace of the daily rhythm in what we do, how we talk and think"

In short, perhaps Tai Chi and Chi Gung can begin to influence our behaviour. By providing slow, rhythmic movement as an object of focus, i.e., instead of an immobile physical posture and static object of focus, the forms give us something to do! Therefore, alongside its health benefits, for those with the potential/inclination, it is perhaps a useful steppingstone for the development of sitting meditation. As Master Da Liu (1974) points out:

"Tai Chi can be considered a kind of preparatory exercise for meditation, although it can be studied for a variety of other reasons. It disciplines the body, teaches relaxation and clear headedness... More than that, Tai Chi Chuan gives something of the spirit of meditation, a spirit which, in our overactive, anxiety ridden

lives, we seldom taste in day to day living – a spirit which promises a glimpse of peace beyond the scope of our present imagination…"

Arguably, sitting meditation pertains more to spiritual development but the main purpose of Tai Chi and Chi Gung, for most people, is perhaps the *"variety of other reasons"* specifically those of physical and mental health. Whichever the case, mindfulness is a necessity for optimum benefit, but it is also to some extent, depending on one's approach, a consequence of the practise of Tai Chi and Chi Gung for health.

So how can we apply mindfulness to the movements of Tai Chi and Chi Gung? In short, one should pay gentle attention to the complete movement and if one becomes distracted, gently bring your attention back to the movement (basic description in earlier chapters). As mentioned earlier (Appendix 5), <u>providing one has had correct training in regulating the breathing</u>, one can learn to coordinate the yin (in) and yang (out) breath with the yin (condensing) and yang (expanding) movement. However, there are some methods which do not require absolute breath coordination but can be practised to useful effect and are conducive to a mindful approach. For example:

1. Commence in the correct sitting or standing posture.
2. Take one, two or three "cleansing breaths". This will start to relax your mind, body, and breath. While doing this, pay attention to maintaining the correct posture.
3. With the final cleansing breath, let your mind "ride the breath" all the way to the dantien (i.e., follow the visualisation of the breath travelling down to just below the navel) and then keep your attention at that point for a while allowing your breath to become relaxed and regular.
4.   As you begin the postures, try to be aware of each stage of the movement without attending to what you have just done or what you are going to do next. Of course, this is only possible once you have learned the movement by heart. Try not to be rigid and tight in your attention, keep light and relaxed and present. When you recognise that you have been distracted, simply let the distraction go and place your attention back on the postures.

5. When you become more adept at the form you are practising, you might try to be aware of how your energy sinks into the root and moves from the root up to the hands (pay attention to the relevant information in the previous chapters, particularly Appendix 7 and Chapter 5) and/or of how the energy of the movement condenses and expands with its yin and yang aspect.

These are just some ways to begin mindfulness in movement. Remember to avoid being overly serious or pensive, keep it light and aware.

APPENDIX 7. RELAXING IN TAI CHI

In Tai Chi and Chi Gung, to be able to correctly generate its natural expanding and condensing movements to useful effect, not only for health but also for those with a martial bent, it is important to be able to relax correctly. Of course, correct training in the methods discussed previously will eventually cause you to arrive at this beneficial state of relaxation. To be able to mobilise the energies of body efficiently and effectively, they must be directed from a clear state of mind, i.e., optimally focused, which is itself relaxed. Through transfer of physical effort within a relaxed and stable body, triggered by a relaxed and stable mind, energy can flow vitally back and forth, in an out, with ease and effect.

From this you might glean that "relaxed" does not mean a state of, practically inert, flaccidity as might occur in sleep or drug induced states or for that matter as seen in some performances of Tai Chi! It is an optimal state of tone wherein it is difficult to identify tension, yet difficult to identify flaccidity. Tai Chi has its own word for this, *sung*. It is not something that can easily be described, it must be experienced through practise but taught by a knowledgeable teacher. To some extent, it can be visualised by watching a good Tai Chi form, not necessarily the graceful but somewhat athletic forms seen in modern Tai Chi competitions. The nature of sung is expressed as being present or relaxed, yet energised, loose and spontaneous.

From sung, directed energies flow outward, freely and uninhibited, yet can readily reverse in response to circumstances. In sung, one feels just right. One can move in response to given conditions and circumstance, the sung of the waist being the arbiter of any response.

Because of sung you should be able to feel the natural ebb and flow of energy or yin-yang as a feeling of condensing (usually accompanying a contracting, inward, closing, or downward movement) and opening (usually accompanying an extending, outward, opening, or upward movement). For more detail on the topic, several authors discuss Yang Chen Fu's 10 principles.

APPENDIX 8. EXERCISE AND BEYOND

The following account is not intended as a substitute for contacting your GP or attending an emergency clinic or following their advice in the event of developing symptoms of disease. It is offered as one example of a basic guide to engender healthy internal and external conditions in order to resist disease states and improve well-being and self-efficacy. Although, its appears extensive, most of the discussion points can easily be condensed and taken on board within normal daily routines without being obsessive. Importantly, it is offered to make living healthier and happier, certainly not to make it miserable.

> ***The best of healers is good cheer***
>
> (Pindarus; c. 518 – 438 BC)

> ***Be relaxed, happy, and without fear…***
>
> (Karma Thinley Rinpoche 1931-)

It can be argued that stress and the anxiety, pensive sadness, and neurosis which arise from it, is a major factor in the development of immune dysfunction and thus limits the ability of the body's defence mechanisms when invaded by pathogenic organisms or assaulted by other disease states. This is clearly evident in the way politicians and hubristic medical/scientific bodies from within their echo-chambers (supported in many cases by celebrities, within their mutual admiration societies) insidiously and palpably to the point of emesis, generate false sentiment, fear and anxiety to promulgate and produce only too willing subjects to achieve their biased and ignorantly short-sighted or perhaps deviously long-sighted goals, resulting in a compliant, dependent, and without doubt (at least from personal observation) mentally and physically unhealthy populace. Regarding health and well-being, such fear and anxiety, etc. has a positive-feedback effect on the induced stress that caused them and further exacerbates diseases - physical and mental - which arise from it**. So, the first order of the day, beyond resisting the influence of professional liars and removing fear and taking control of one's own destiny and health, is to try to reduce stress and emphasise activities that will prevent its initial assault and reduce or eliminate its effects, e.g., meditation, regular efficacious exercise, healthy diet/lifestyle, appropriately timed remedial action, and a personally relevant spiritual emphasis.

The introductory quotations above might be perceived as trite but nevertheless, they emphasise a state of mind that has very profound effects on health and so it might be best, in the first instance, to make a stab at that.

So, for what it is worth, here are some suggestions that briefly elaborate some actions that might contribute to *"good cheer"* and to *"being relaxed and happy"* and help the body to adapt to pathogenic assault, consequently become stronger as a result (in most cases) and, desirably, resist disease conditions without succumbing to serious adverse effects. These methods and other balanced approaches to health and wellbeing, notwithstanding the pharmaceutical manipulation of microorganisms and molecules to produce substances that promise to save us from disease and death, provide us with mechanisms whereby individuals can create conditions conducive to optimal health and immune function. These preventive and reactive strategies are nothing new, as we can glean from the ancient text *The Yellow Emperor's Classic of Internal Medicine*.

The Yellow Emperor once inquired of his ministers:

"I've heard that in days of old everyone lived over one hundred years without showing the usual signs of aging. In our time however, people age prematurely… Is it due to a change in environment or is it because people have lost the correct way of life?"

Qi Bo the chief physician answered:

"In the past… people understood the principle of yin and yang balance… These days, people have changed their way of life. They drink wine as though it were water, indulge excessively in destructive activities, that drain their body's essence and deplete their vital force… Seeking emotional excitement and momentary pleasures, people disregard the natural rhythm and order of the universe. They fail to regulate their lifestyle and diet, and sleep improperly… Internally, they are enslaved by their emotions and worries. They work too hard in heavy labour.

(Maoshing Ni, 1995)

Sound familiar? Without ruminating on the nature of moral behaviour and the characteristics of hedonism, I think that what we can extract from Qi Bo's assessment, if we are to maintain good health, is the need for a more regulated lifestyle that avoids extremes and excesses. Despite the many health interventions available to us, the most important way for humans to resist pathogenic influences, such as environmental factors, viruses, and bacteria, or at least ameliorate the severity of their adverse effects and aid recovery once affected, is to adopt a personally responsible, more measured, harmonious, and natural lifestyle.

The following suggests a balanced approach to some important aspects of lifestyle and health (not including specific and necessary therapeutic treatments) that has to some extent stood me in good stead over the years, along with my family and past patients. I am certain that it is not perfect or definitive and that there are other views and approaches that might be more specific or superior but not necessarily achievable for some of us at this point in time. It is not meant as medical advice for specific illnesses, although it might well help when used in conjunction with the guidance of appropriate health-care professionals such as doctors, nurses, herbalists, etc. It is what I consider, from personal experience, to be part of a balanced, pro-active approach to health maintenance. It is a proactive approach which the ancient physician Qi Bo (2500BCE) alludes to when he states, *"To take medicine when you are sick is like digging a well only when you are thirsty - is it not already too late?"*

A general approach to supporting health and well-being.
The reader might be wondering why I included a general section on health in a book about Tai Chi and Chi Gung (Chinese exercise methods, adapted in part from martial systems). I have done so because, in a pro-active approach to health, it is not enough to exercise without attending to other essential necessities for health. As with Chi Gung exercise, one should maintain a balanced approach and avoid obsession, excesses, or indulgence in narcissistic fads. As Qi Bo informs the Yellow Emperor:

"In ancient times, people lived simply......When the weather was cooled, they became active to fend off the cold. When the weather heated up in summer, they retreated to cool places. Internally their emotions were calm and peaceful, they were

without excessive desires. Externally they did not have the stress of today. They lived without greed and desire... They maintained inner peace and concentration of mind and spirit. This prevented pathogens from invading.... When they did contract disease, they simply guided properly their emotions and spirit and redirected the energy flow using the method of zhou you [treatment]."

(Maoshing Ni, 1995)

For convenience, we might say there are two general categories of approach that should be encouraged in a balanced approach to health. The first and unquestionably most important is, as the ancient physician Qi Bo often implies, a "pro-active" approach, which refers to encouraging a healthy internal environment (and sound structural support) within a healthy as possible external environment that *"prevents pathogens invading"* (this might imply any disease state). The second is the "re-active" approach, which refers to addressing the problem after it has occurred and usually when it is acute or has become chronic, i.e., *"using the method of zhou you"*. However, although it is useful to discuss healthcare in terms of these two categories, they are not disparate, as the distinction between proactive and reactive often depends on when and how the methods are utilised. For example, pro-active methods such as Chi Gung and massage, can also be used to treat disease once it has taken hold and reactive methods such as some medicines, herbs and nutrition can be used to prevent disease occurring. Nevertheless, the pro-active view and approach is most prudent. The following story told by Liang and Wu (1993) illustrates the superior nature of pro-active healthcare and, dare I suggest, a reason why there is more of an emphasis on reactive healthcare in the West!

There were once three brothers who were all doctors. The first could repair major damage and so received gifts and adulation from his patients. His fame spread far and wide as his skills were easily noticeable. The second brother could cure disease before it resulted in major damage, so his fame was great but not as extensive as the first brother. He was known only in his region. The third brother was hardly known, yet his skill was the greatest of all! Of all three, the brother who was the least known was the greatest (but perhaps the poorest) because his methods (Chi Gung) prevented disease before it occurred, i.e., a pro-active approach! Oh well, to borrow from Queen, we can't all have, *"fame and fortune and everything that goes with it"*!

Why a Pro-active approach?

It is desirable to adopt a realistic (and therefore, manageable) and even-minded approach (i.e., avoiding a narcissistic or obsessive approach) to your own welfare and be actively involved in programmes that will engender continued well-being or recovery from disease. In this process, the aid of doctors, nurses, and other healthcare folk, of any reputable tradition, cannot be dismissed, but unless medical intervention becomes necessary, it is preferable that they should only provide support and encouragement for a pro-active approach to repair and maintenance. The pro-active approach supports nature in what it does best, when allowed to do so. As Voltaire is reputed to have pointed out *"The art of medicine consists in amusing the patient while nature cures the disease"*. Somewhat humorous, shallow, and limited in view, but you perhaps get at least one allusion that not uncommonly, given the right conditions, our bodies will naturally function effectively with little or no external intervention (review introductory note).

The inception and development of public health and welfare systems has of course brought many benefits, not otherwise available to a natural/traditional approach to health. It is therefore unfortunate (and perhaps ironic) that it has, perhaps inadvertently, fostered a mistaken, over-reliant "cradle to grave" mentality and instead of promoting "freedom from fear" (quote used slightly out of context for effect) has created an atmosphere and conditions that blatantly promote fear and sadly entitlement. Furthermore, instead of developing a healthy community, it seems to have engendered a default acceptable epidemic of chronic and acute poor health (self-induced or otherwise). We appear to be tolerating poor health and perhaps this is partly because we have become over-reliant on our healthcare professionals (many of whom are well-intentioned and wonderful; some, not so much) whom we obsequiously and over-sentimentally applaud in times of need, but when the sentiment wanes are only too ready to criticise and even draw into litigation! Bless them and keep them safe from such meanness and hypocrisy. It is perhaps worth remembering, when we put these people on pedestals, the biblical warning of *awesome* golden idols having *feet of clay*, then perhaps we might not be so reliant upon them and at least we might be more understanding and forgiving when they err. I digress!

There are many reasons for our epidemic of poor health but no doubt a mindset of abnegation of personal-responsibly for one's own health is a major factor. Strongly complicit in this is a wilful ignoring or rejection of preventive/pro-active strategies, which is in no small part due to relinquishing of our knowledge of fundamental principles of health with the consequent over-dependence on allopathic medicine to extricate us from our, often, self-inflicted conditions. Consider the wonderful manifestation of a caring society, the National Health Service; arguably, mismanaged and unquestionably abused, battling to stay afloat amongst an over-reliant populace with unrealistic expectations of the medical profession (and perhaps a medical profession with a "magnificent obsession" that sometimes results in a well-meaning but deluded view of the superiority and efficacy of their own methods and wares). In the aforementioned mindset of abnegation and dependence, when illness or the fear of illness manifests, it can be very tempting to fully relinquish personal responsibility and hand over the reins to a professional "saviour" (which they often are) who, with the best of intentions, will take you where they think you need to go (or even where they think you think you need to go!). It is far more empowering and self-efficacious in the long term if you keep one hand on the reins in situations concerning yourself. Of course, it will occasionally and inevitably be expedient and necessary to engage with your medical advisor (allopathic, surgical, herbal, or otherwise). In these cases, you must "assume that the person you are listening to might know something [beyond Google!] you don't" (Peterson, 2018) - wise advice in more than just health care. However, with deep gratitude and a fond adieu, you should re-take the reins at your earliest but medically appropriate convenience.

When a Re-active approach?
When illness takes hold, a reactive approach should be appropriately timed. To reiterate, seek and accept help when you need it, the earlier the better. We are very fortunate to live in a society where there are skilled and compassionate individuals (in all their wonderful manifestations) who have worked hard at great personal and financial expense to develop their skills and knowledge (yes, beyond Google!)

and have perhaps experienced some of the many ailments that arise from simply being human. They can often help directly (by medical, physical, psychological, and emotional interventions), or at least "point the way". However, to reiterate Qi Bo's warning: "*To take medicine when you are sick is like digging a well only when you are thirsty - is it not already too late?*" alluding to the sanity of a pro-active approach. So now I will highlight some elements of a pro-active approach.

Under the heading of pro-action, we can consider three appropriate methods: appropriate activity, appropriate diet, and appropriate remedies - i.e., using them in a preventative way.

1. Appropriate activity

The physician Sun Si Miao explained, '*Moving water does not stagnate, active hinges never rust*'. While one can interpret his metaphor in varying depth, we can simply say that lack of movement results in stagnation and of course, stagnation inevitably results in conditions, environmental and physiological, conducive to pathogenic/disease states, e.g. abnormal tissue states (referring specifically to understanding of the quality and activity of organs etc.); energy stagnation or excess - inhibited or excessive neural (nervous system), humoral (immune system and hormones), fluid (circulation/chi), joint (skeleton) and tissue activity (muscles and organs); inappropriate absorption (how well we absorb nutrients) and elimination (how well we remove waste), etc. The optimal activity of these systems is vital for maintaining and improving health and as mentioned earlier, all pro-active and re-active methods should consider all these points and, importantly, how they affect and are affected by our mental state, e.g., stress and anxiety, etc.

Regular exercise, especially slow, rhythmic, condensing and expanding movement, encourages effective internal stimulation of tissues and movement of fluids. With regard to reduction of stress, anxiety, etc., exercise should be also directed toward gently and progressively strengthening the constitution in order to gain physical and emotional strength and self-efficacy and further help to resist pathogenic influence. To this end, as indicated in the main text, exercises collectively known as Chi Gung are extremely effective. Not only does Chi Gung address the physical necessities to engender healthy tissues, it utilises natural breathing techniques, postures and movement to develop mindfulness and clarity (something which is commonly lost to the overactive mind of stress and anxiety, which can often degenerate into the melancholic pensiveness of depression) and invigorates the spirit. Correct posture is a profound basis for Chi Gung effectiveness and for that matter all aspects of physiological and mental health.

Why is correct posture important?

Initially, for some, the corrective basic posture of Chi Gung is a somewhat contrived physical act of emerging from low spirits and beginning to address the depressed or maladjusted physical and mental constitution. How so? By a determined, "active reversal process". Why and how does this help? Consider that the state of our mind is often reflected in the way we hold ourselves - this is a manifest "mind-body" effect. For example, when we feel healthy and in good spirits, we might display an open and raised countenance. On the other hand, if we are depressed, we might be stooped, folding into ourselves, and then perhaps become caught up in a positive-feedback loop where the depression gets worse and then, too often, we can become susceptible to other illnesses. What is to be done in this case, how can we begin to apply an "active reversal process"? We can, where possible, utilise the opposite "body-mind" effect, i.e., the theory that physical /physiological conditions affect the state of mind. In this case, beneficially adjusting the physical, will beneficially affect the state of the mind.

Why should this be the case? Consider how you feel when you have a physical/painful injury. Are you mentally in a good place? Unlikely! What happens to your mental state when the pain is prolonged? Perhaps you might find it difficult to cope psychologically/emotionally as well as physically and even become depressed, etc. What happens to your mental state when the pain is relieved, pharmaceutically, or otherwise? Perhaps you become less adversely affected psychologically and emotionally. In both cases the physical state has to some degree affected the state of mind. There are complex mechanisms involved and I have oversimplified them here but there is no question, now even in the modern medical model (i.e., "functional medicine"), that our mental state affects the physical state and vice-versa.

So then, to affect the state of mind beneficially, whether for maintaining physical health or helping to improve our mental state *per se* we can at least make a start by adjusting body structure, often to noticeable effect. The clinical psychologist Jordan Peterson (2018) advises (or perhaps admonishes), *"…attend carefully to your posture. Quit drooping and hunching around… walk tall and gaze forthrightly ahead… Encourage the serotonin* [a brain chemical that affects mood] *to flow plentifully through the neural pathways desperate for its calming influence"*. Could it be that when we adopt or, initially, just simulate this correct (and corrective) posture found in Chi Gung, we are imitating what we often do naturally when we "lift ourselves out of the doldrums" or when we are about to embark upon a difficult task that perhaps we are unsure of achieving and so we are, perhaps, causing the *"serotonin to flow plentifully"*. Naturally, we often tend to, if not totally overwhelmed by fear and anxiety, "soldier on" by lifting the head and body upward to raise our spirits and expand our physical presence so that we can engage the task with some courage and confidence (a countenance which is sadly diminishing in the developing environments of mask-wearing). Thus, we engage with our surroundings while being mindful of our task instead of closing down and pensively mulling over the situation. Even if somewhat feigned at first, adopting this posture eventually may become a good habit, which can then become natural and thus, efficacious in the long term. To borrow a Buddhist analogy, in order to straighten a bent arrow, you first need to bend it in the other direction. So too, we may initially have to force or feign correct posture to overcome any habitual tendency or entrenched distortion. I am not suggesting that this physical action is the perfect way for everyone to feel better, but it might be a good start for some. Clearly, there is more to health and well-being than just correct posture, but it is an important starting point. As mentioned, correct posture is a profound basis for good mental and physical health. Therefore, methods that develop or encourage a raised and open posture with a strong foundation, such as Tai Chi and Chi Gung, Yoga, the Alexander method, etc. are indispensable in a pro-active approach to health.

At the risk of rambling, but for completeness, it is worth mentioning the "body-body" effect, a term which can be used to describe how any bodily dysfunction, especially if unresolved, can result in a reflex dysfunction in other parts of the body. As we are discussing posture, a perhaps banal example is the nerve compression caused by incorrect or abnormal structure of the spine, which results in pain and wasting of the muscles that the motor nerve innervates. Clearly, a dysfunction in one part of the body, the spine, affects another part, a muscle. So, by applying or developing appropriate adjustment or readjustment of incorrect structure we can surely beneficially affect another part of the body. Extending this example of nerve compression caused by structural abnormality, by correcting structure we can remove the offending compression and thus, the wasting muscle can be correctly innervated and nourished to return to health. However, attention must also be paid to the distal problem if one wishes to fully address the "ostensive" cause.

The point to be emphasised here is that for any problem to be fully addressed, all three reflex mechanisms should be considered and a key element central to all three interactions is that of correct structure/posture. I should also point out that in addition to such active methods as Tai Chi, etc., there are also passive modalities, in the form of manipulation and massage that can contribute to not only structural but visceral and even psychological health. Importantly, referring to my critique of our situation of community poor health, bear in mind that for all these methods to be effective, the will to address one's problems and help oneself needs to be present.

With correct posture in mind, in a pro-active approach to health and well-being, one should endeavour to carry out regular, safe, non-competitive exercise. Although, there is nothing particularly wrong with competitive exercise *per se* (although excessive exercise can adversely affect immune function) that is another story, and this is about optimum health, not being the best or developing the "body-beautiful". We have seen that in addition to ensuring effective movement, non-competitive exercise can reduce and perhaps neutralise the effects of the often connected and synergistic pathogenic conditions of depression/anxiety and stress and their concomitant morbidities. Recalling the advice of Nyanaponika Mahathera:

"To counter the unhealthy effects of the frantic pace of modern life, it is imperative that, in our free time, we try consciously to pause and slow down...

slowing down is helpful in reducing mental and physical tension... Beyond the immediate effects of an exercise session, slowing down exercises influence the pace of the daily rhythm in what we do, how we talk and think".

Of course, I am labouring the point that a unique and comprehensive set of exercises which meet these criteria can be found in the Chinese methods of Tai Chi and Chi Gung but as mentioned, other methods can be utilised effectively to a greater or lesser degree. As my friend, retired psychology lecturer and unrepentant athlete, John Pouncy, pointed out to me recently *"Solvitur ambulando et currendo"*, which I think, loosely translated, implies we can overcome our problems by walking and running - sound advice. However, in deference to my own tradition, the apparently effortless, rhythmic postures and associated mindfulness, encourage harmony of mind, body, and vital energy (known as *Chi* in Chinese medical theory) to engender a state of mental and physical well-being. To reiterate from the Yellow Emperor's Classic of Internal Medicine:

"When internal energies are able to circulate smoothly and freely, and the energy of the mind is not scattered, but focused and concentrated, illness and disease can be avoided"

To consolidate my laboured emphasis, a unique aspect of Chi Gung is that, unlike other forms of exercise, it is not limited by the weather, time, or space (perfect in the current state of confinement), and because it does not rely on strength, speed or prowess, it can be enjoyed by people of all abilities, age and gender; anywhere, anytime!

Activity in Fresh Air and Sunlight

Last, but not only and not least, with regard to appropriate activity, it is essential that we get out in the fresh air, into open, green spaces and natural light (Just in case you need science, some research suggests this has a beneficial effect on the immune system ☺). We are, at least in a molecular sense, a synthesis of these conditions, so it is reasonable to assume that appropriate exposure to such an environment will nourish us. Conversely, the further we remove ourselves from that environment, the less we will be nourished. As Carl Sagan pointed out *"We are all connected: to each other biologically; to the earth chemically; and to the rest of the universe atomically"* An important element of our locale of the biological and chemical "universe", that is essential to our survival and that of the planet which supports and nourishes us, is of course the Sun and its energy. Therefore, for a variety of reasons, not least of all resistance to infectious disease, it is important that we have access, wherever possible, to natural light and the natural, open, clean air spaces that have themselves resulted from its nourishing energies. Although the detail of this topic is beyond the scope of this brief essay, you should pay attention to the importance of sunlight and health (for a useful starting point see Hobday, 1999). In any event, whenever you can, get out into the fresh air, preferably near a nice big tree and practise your Tai Chi, meditation or exercise, there is nothing like it!

Finally, take a trip to town and have a large chocolate and caramel latte (its healthy because it contains vanilla and cinnamon sprinkles), and a cheese (full of calcium) and bacon (great source of protein) toastie (digestible carbs), topping it off with a healthy, glucose-fructose syrup sweetened, gluten free brownie… Ha-ha, just joking! Talking about diet…

2. Appropriate Diet

One should always consider one's individual medical history regarding food intolerance, allergies, etc. However, appropriate diet is nothing more, or less, than ensuring appropriate and effective nourishment for mind and body and by virtue of that, spirit.

In Brief:
- Other than special therapeutic dietary needs, maintain a balanced diet. Avoid processed food.
- Do not eat too much of anything at one time.
- Eat plenty of colourful, fresh fruit and vegetables and incorporate healthy herbs and spices.
- Keep Hydrated. Drink sufficient water, as pure and natural as you can get it.
- If you are vegetarian, make sure you have complete nutrition, even more so if you are vegan, as these diets do not have the easy access to essential proteins, fats, vitamins, and minerals readily found in meats.

- If you eat meat, try to avoid excess. If possible, source it as 'free from' as you can (free from substances antithetical to health – there are lots of them about!).

- If you eat raw wholefoods, that is good; especially when you are trying to address a particular health issue, but cooked/hot food is necessary, and more effectively digested

- KEEP IT MOVING! It is important to have sufficient wholesome fibre in your diet. If you do not pooh easily and regularly, then something is amiss in your lifestyle and/or diet.

- When you decide to eat, EAT - do not multitask, it is not a virtue! i.e., sit down, enjoy, and digest the food – respect it, it was hard come-by!

- Enjoy the things you like but in moderation - unless it causes intolerance, allergy, or reactive conditions.

- Regular supplements are an important part of a daily health regimen, especially in these times of forced, nutritionally deficient and ultra-processed food sources.

In more detail:

Adopt a straightforward, balanced approach to a diet that avoids extremes or faddish ideas. If attended to in a measured manner, appropriate diet will surely prove efficacious. The following are general safe guidelines; try your best to work towards them. However, a word of warning, they are not a substitute for medical dietary advice or necessary medical treatments. Also, if you have a specific condition, consult a relevant medical professional before embarking upon any special dietary or exercise programme.

To emphasise, avoid fad diets. Even before the advent of the internet, one person or another with their, arguably, narrow, and pedantic world view, presented, what they no doubt thought, sound reasons for criticising existing nutritional theories in favour of their own. They may or may not have validity but for sure, sooner or later, someone else will come along and put paid to their theories with a newer, more "valid" theory! Many people will undoubtedly swear by this new or old or whatever diet for one reason or another, but they may be trading short-term gains for long-term problems if the diet lacks appropriate balance. In the health arena, there are several views and rationale with regard to sources and ratios of nutrients but for the generally healthy individual, without nutrient related pathologies and intolerances, keeping your diet roughly within the range of the WHO recommendations (I am not an advocate for WHO!) for daily nutrient intake is probably a useful and appropriate but very general starting point, e.g. 55-75% carbohydrates (Here, I am referring mostly to unrefined carbs e.g. vegetables, etc); 10-15% protein (meat, pulses, eggs etc.); 15-30% fats (saturated fats are important but one should ensure a proportion of fats are from unsaturated fats from oils, etc.); sugary substances less than 10% - much less! (These should be unrefined, and their sweetness derived largely from an unprocessed source). I tend to be more definite about dietary ratios than WHO as I am not particularly concerned with the enormous profits made from pushing excess intake of sugar, meat, and animal/saturated fats. Not that, arguably, there is anything inherently bad about these foods, other than over-indulgence, excess and addiction; however, I only ever suggest what I know to have been beneficial for myself, my family and past patients.

Carbohydrate sources

- Try to eat up to around five servings a day of dark green, leafy and root vegetables, e.g., broccoli, cabbage, sprouts, carrots, parsnips, green beans, salad greens, peppers etc. (Yes, some of these foods do contain "adverse nutrients" but in a balanced diet, especially if cooked properly, for individuals who are not predisposed to certain conditions, the adverse effects are often irrelevant).

- Try to eat a minimum of three servings of fresh fruit or more a day, e.g., apples, pears, berries, citrus fruit, etc. These are best eaten raw, but sometimes it is useful to apply "mechanical mastication" or heat, especially when trying to nourish poorly folk.

- Incorporate whole grains into your diet (unless you have a problem with them), e.g., whole grain rice, whole oats, pulses, quinoa, etc. If you are not intolerant to wheat which contain insoluble fibre and is high in gluten (lots of people are intolerant, to a greater or lesser degree) you can incorporate whole-wheat bread in reasonable amounts. Individuals who must contend with bowel disorders such as IBS, might need to utilise soluble fibre foods but it is best to consult an appropriate health practitioner about this (e.g., a doctor, herbalist, naturopath, nutritionist, etc.).

- Avoid refined sugar (even the packs that say unrefined or at least reduce intake, i.e., of white OR brown. Glucose-Fructose syrup (in all its guises) has been shown to be NOT good - that's all I am going to say about that ☺! Avoid artificial sweeteners – they are probably not helpful – do your own research (There is a suggestion that Stevia is useful, but the jury is still out). If you do need to sweeten your foods (and you usually don't) use <u>small amounts</u> of unprocessed honey (it has some useful beneficial effects) or other unprocessed sweeteners that contain nutritionally useful substances. If you are interested in the sugar issue, and it is a big issue, you might wish to read "Pure, White and Deadly: How Sugar Is Killing Us and What We Can Do to Stop It" (Yudkin, 2016). Although I am banging on about sugar, it important to have balance, and the occasional treat is fine and can in fact be beneficial to one's demeanour! It's a cost-benefit thing! ☺

- Avoid sugary drinks and carbonated drinks. Most concentrated fruit juices are "done to death" and are basically sugary fluid, so you should dilute them (when we eat the whole fruits, we absorb the sugars less rapidly along with other vital nutrients and our body has to work to digest and assimilate them). If you must have sweet drinks, freshly "juiced" fruits and veg juices or freshly made "rainbow food" smoothies ('mechanically masticated') are preferable.

Protein sources

- If you are an omnivore, it is all about balance and not eating meat (or anything) in excessive amounts. Although there is a strong moral argument against eating animal flesh, it is not particularly unhealthy (except for the animal who was killed) to eat meat and fat as some might have you believe. So, notwithstanding ethical considerations, if you have a high intake of red meat, reduce it, and perhaps replace it with white meat, fish, and oily fish. I am not personally recommending it, it's up to you! I should highlight that I cannot speak for some dietary approaches that emphasise a higher meat intake.

- If you are vegetarian, that is a healthy way to live, PROVIDING YOU MAINTAIN A BALANCED DIET (some "unaware" vegetarians do not). You should ensure you eat a variety of vegetable proteins in place of meat proteins, e.g. As a suggestion, try to eat two servings of beans, lentils, or fermented soya (e.g., natto, tempeh and miso) each day. There are others but you should avoid focussing on just one type.

- If you are not vegan, then eggs are an excellent source of nutrients (despite the, I believe, biased demonisation of cholesterol), including proteins, vitamins, and minerals. True free-range eggs (free to roam and forage on pastures) are perhaps the better option. Even better if they are organic.

Fat sources

- Saturated fats are an important part of our nutritional requirements but should be used appropriately (this topic is controversial regarding heart disease, etc. – do your own research). Unless you are vegetarian, saturated fats can be obtained from meat but is also sourced from coconut oil, butter etc. Avoid foods containing hydrogenated/trans-fats, e.g., found in some spreads, and pastries etc.

- Unless you are vegan, dairy products can be a useful and satiating dietary source but avoid excessive intake. Avoid them altogether if you are intolerant or allergic to them. A useful milk substitute might be almond, oat or rice milk (but they take a little getting used to and should not be overused as I have no doubt that some adverse-effect or other will be highlighted in the future!). There is some, not invalid, controversy about the adverse effects of unfermented soy products so excessive use of unfermented soya milk as a milk replacement might not be a useful strategy – do your own research!

- Try to incorporate into your diet foods containing important essential fats, e.g., foods such as walnuts, pumpkin seeds, sunflower seeds, etc. (Grind up a tablespoon and sprinkle onto your breakfast cereal, or salad). Oily fish are an important source of healthy essential fat.

- Natural probiotic yoghurt or similar fermented product (as opposed to just a plain dairy yoghurt) is beneficial to digestion and the digestive system and a useful source of fats, carbs, proteins, vitamins, and minerals. It is an excellent topping for fresh fruits (although there might be some debate about this combination, particularly in Ayurveda, I have not noted any problems other than in some individuals with certain digestive issues). You could add a sprinkle of your favourite muesli or ground seeds and a good dash of cinnamon or mixed spice for flavour (and to aid physiological functions).

It is worth reiterating the point here about fad diets, this includes in vogue ideas overconfidently promoted by medics, which, vicariously, carry the qualification of science, but, as with much science theory, once research is extended, it is found to be flawed or lacking. Regarding fats etc., and prevention of cardiovascular disease, a humorous parody, of an old rhyme, attributed to the great pioneer heart surgeon Christiaan Barnard, warned against eggs, and saturated fats:

> *Early to bed, early to rise, take non-competitive exercise.*
> *Avoid all stress, take care not to eat, eggs, butter, cheese, and meat.*
> *That it is bad to be male has been clearly proved, so have your*
> *testicles removed!*

Some valid points, but wrong in so many ways ☺. So, I think I will stick to the original adage:

> *Early to bed, early to rise, makes a man healthy, wealthy, and wise.*

Fluid intake
- Drink plenty of fluid throughout the day (it is important not to drink too much, too fast). Two litres of fluid is thought to provide an appropriate volume for the average adult in the average day, at least half of which should be pure water. Everything important

that happens in our body happens in a fluid environment that is water-based, it is required in optimum amount for things to work properly. Dehydration is not always clinically apparent, and our bodies learn to adapt to "sub-clinical" dehydration, which can manifest as cravings for food and stimulants such as coffee and sweet stuff. This type of dehydration can result in general feelings of malaise or a vague feeling of being unwell to a variety of illnesses. So why not eliminate dehydration and feel generally better by ensuring you drink enough water. Avoid, at least too much, consumption of too cold water - room temperature or warm is perhaps best (yes, enjoy the occasional cold drink - live a little ☺). NB Care should be taken not to over hydrate as in certain individuals this can adversely affect electrolyte levels and water retention issues. For purpose of digestion, it might be best not to drink too much water when eating a meal. If you need to, then just take small sips.

- Avoid drinking excess coffee and tea. Although they have some useful and beneficial effects, relatively large amounts can exacerbate anxiety and stress and cause difficulty sleeping, which is essential to a healthy mind, body, and immune system. They are diuretic in nature and if you tend not to drink water, they can cause chronic or sub-clinical dehydration. However, green tea is useful for a variety of health reasons, depending on the type. You can vary your beverages by replacing tea and coffee with healthy herb teas (see 3 Appropriate Remedies). It is beneficial to drink water on rising as we tend to dehydrate overnight and tea and coffee first thing, although, stimulating, might later in the day result in tiredness, etc.

- Avoid sweetened drinks such as cola, especially diet sodas and fizzy drinks. They contain the ideal ingredient for making human lard: sugar! Drinks with artificial sweeteners are suspect from a health perspective and are associated with increased appetite and consequent unhelpful weight gain. For sweet drinks, it is best to make your own fresh juice or smoothie. Again, balance is the key, enjoying the odd fizzy drink will not generally be bad for you. However, swilling it down every day from the cheap multipack and giant bottles pushed without shame but voluntarily purchased in large quantities from discount stores and supermarkets, will certainly contribute to obesity and consequent poor health.

General

- For a variety of reasons avoid heavily processed foods. Processing reduces the effective nutritional value and can cause poor digestion and elimination deficits. In addition, some research shows they can affect the immune system adversely.

- Despite misinformed and constant ridicule by the orthodox medical profession (less so of late), it is useful to take certain nutritional supplements. Supplementation is something that we need to be wary of with regards to what is or is not useful as this is also subject to fads and trends, so it is worthwhile obtaining advice from a reputable and experienced practitioner (e.g., a herbalist or naturopath, nutritionist etc.). However, a useful general daily supplement programme should at least incorporate a multivitamin/mineral. Avoid poor quality supplements that you might find in some stores and ensure you purchase supplements of good quality that the body can absorb and assimilate optimally. I prefer a brand of "Food-State" supplements - you can purchase these or other good quality supplements from a reputable health food shop. The use of therapeutic doses of vitamins such as C, D3, etc., to enhance immune function and resist infectious disease, can be quite specific relating to age, size, etc. and so best undertaken with advice from a relevant qualified practitioner.

- Take regular exercise. You guessed it, Tai Chi and Chi Gung, or walking, running (appropriate to your level), swimming, cycling, dancing, etc. are all excellent forms of exercise (but make sure it is within your physical capability). These things are essential to healthy digestion but also help maintain healthy functioning of mind and body, to lift one's spirit, and engender a feeling of well-being, which is especially important to immune function.

- Try to relax. Regarding diet, it will certainly aid digestion and elimination. In any case, it is useful to learn and practise relaxation-meditation techniques, Yoga or Tai Chi/Chi Gung.

Stress is a major factor in digestive disease development and progression. These methods, by their very nature, help to engender a mindful approach to eating in addition to our general situation. They create the ideal conditions for digestive processes and if nothing else provide a brief and enjoyable respite from our problems throughout the day. It is worth mentioning that a wholesome, personally appropriate, spiritual path and practice is essential not only to one's spiritual welfare, but also to well-being of mind and body.

- Extending the point on relaxation, recall *"early to bed, early to rise…"*; like *"good cheer"*, sleep is a great healer. Sufficed to say that enough sleep and not too much is necessary to ensure optimal physiological and psychological/emotional health. The issue is complex, particularly with regard to insomnia and so it is important, if you are having such problems, to try and establish the cause. In general, however, one should avoid becoming involved in complex mental activity or problem solving prior to bedtime and avoid staying up late watching disturbingly violent and horrific programmes, such as the news ☺. Do something which helps you "switch off". Where possible, switch off or block all lighting, even mobile charging lights etc. and block out or dampen street lighting. If needed for personal/safety reasons, it might be best to use a soft, warm nightlight (not an open-lit candle – for safety reasons).

3. Appropriate Remedies

Proactive methods are vital to our health and well-being. They are generally safe and effective but sometimes, despite our best efforts, things can go wrong (that's life!). When this occurs, you should always seek advice from an appropriate medical professional - the sooner, the better. Natural treatment is a preferable option (e.g., herbalist /naturopath) but not always appropriate, orthodox treatment (e.g., GP, etc.) is necessary in acute or potentially acute conditions. The ancient physician Sun Simiao offers some definitive guidance:

"First, modify the patient's diet and lifestyle and only then, if these do not effect a cure, treat with medicinals and acupuncture".

In any event, a competent and qualified practitioner will know their limitations and refer appropriately.

Professional consultation notwithstanding, to try to help reduce the need for medical intervention we should also take the pro-active approach to "remedies" as suggested in this section of a clever ditty attributed to David Paul Brown – whoever, he was! (From the North American Magazine, 1883):

> '*Let doctors or quacks prescribe as they may,*
> *Yet none of their nostrums for me;*
> *For I firmly believe-what the old women say-*
> *That there's nothing like camomile tea.*
>
> *It strengthens the mind, it enlivens the brain,*
> *It converts all our sorrow to glee;*
> *It heightens our pleasures, it banishes pain-*
> *Then what is like camomile tea?*
>
> *In health, it is harmless-and, say what you please,*
> *One thing is still certain with me,*
> *It suits equally well with every disease;*
> *Oh, there's nothing like camomile tea.*'

Whether you like or dislike chamomile tea, implicit in these verses is the proactive and reactive nature of such remedies. The function of remedies (in the proactive sense) is dietary, yet they should gently but profoundly affect mind, body and, when used in conjunction with appropriate activity and diet, indirectly affect spirit. For an appropriate and proactive health remedy, there is nothing like chamomile tea of course (except for those with an allergy to the *Compositae* family of plants, to which it belongs)! For the dis-likers of chamomile, there are many other herbs that can be safely used for such purposes, many (including chamomile) are used by Herbalists to enhance immune function and recovery from infection. Several herbs can safely be used to enhance general health some can be pleasantly used to replace tea and coffee (which are themselves traditional herbal remedies). You can find a selection of these in *National Institute of Medical Herbalist* publications and many excellent books written by its members. See appendix seven for some useful herbs recommended by NIMH.

Herbs can of course be utilised effectively in the treatment of many illnesses, but it is best to consult a qualified Herbalist, Homoeopath or Naturopath on such matters. For details of highly trained and qualified Medical Herbalists see www.nimh.org.uk

*** For more a more in-depth discussion of stress regarding health see Understanding Chi Kung by John and Peter Farrell*

APPENDIX 9. A SUMMARY OF SOME USEFUL AND SUPPORTIVE HERB TEAS

I have included this list of useful herbs for health that help to keep things moving. They are also useful those who might be interested in occasional alternatives to tea and coffee. Many teas can be purchased as loose herb or in teabags. Some herbs, like foods and other medicines do not always agree with some constitutions or disease states, so they should be avoided in such cases. If uncertain as to whether they are safe for you, obtain advice from your local Medical Herbalist. As always, if you do use herbs for tisanes, moderation is the key.

This information is taken directly from a free NIMH leaflet and slightly adapted by the author.

Cardamom fruit - relieves flatulence, harmonises digestion and eases nausea. Useful for combating colds and chills.

Celery seed - A cleansing herb, offering a good source of minerals, beneficial for kidneys and frequently used for joint disorders. Avoid in pregnancy.

Chamomile flowers - The 'mother of the gut'. Used for digestive weakness. Also, very helpful to alleviate tension. A pleasant herb for children, to relieve colic and promote rest. Add an infusion to your bath. Use as a final rinse for your hair.

Cinnamon quills - A herb to aid the circulation, promote good digestion, and to help combat infection. Avoid in pregnancy.

Dandelion root/leaf - Frequently used to reduce water retention (oedema). High in minerals which are frequently depleted by synthetic diuretics. Seek help from you GP or herbalist if you suffer from water retention

Elderflower - A lovely tasting tea, generally used to relieve cold symptoms, including catarrh and sinus problems. Can be used to make a lovely wine or cordial.

Fennel seed - a digestive agent to help relieve griping and indigestion. Encourages milk supply when breastfeeding. Useful herb to relieve colic in children.

Ginger root and stem – a carminative used to ease digestive discomfort and nausea. It is beneficial for poor circulation. In feverish conditions it promotes perspiration. Pleasant when taken with lemon and other spices such as cinnamon.

Lemon balm herb - A refreshing, gentle herb to relieve anxiety, promote digestion and induce rest. Has antiviral activity.

Lemon verbena herb - similar activities to lemon balm, but with a slightly different flavour.

Limeflower - Another anti-stress herb for soothing the nervous system. Used by herbalists for some individuals with high blood pressure and circulatory disorders. Consult you GP or herbalist if you suffer from circulatory disorders.

Marigold flowers - A cleansing, detoxifying herb with antifungal and antibiotic activity. Marigold exhibits these properties internally and externally. Use as a wash, compress, foot, and hip bath.

Nettle herb - No wonder this herb is so widely available, it is very good for us! A detoxifier that traditionally was used as a spring tonic. Herbalists use this for a wide range of conditions, including allergies and joint disorders, Use nettles in soups with other vegetables. A good hair tonic, (Use in the final rinse).

Peppermint herb - a herb for the digestive system having stimulant properties. Harmonises well with elderflower for colds and catarrh. Try peppermint to relieve headaches. Maximum of 4 cups per day. Do not use for children under four. Makes a pleasant foot bath. Avoid if suffering from reflux disease.

Rosemary herb - encourages digestive function. Traditionally used to increase circulation to the head, relieve pain and enhance concentration. Maximum 3 cups per day. Do not use if you have high blood pressure.

Sage herb - Useful anti-infective herb. Excellent as a gargle to relieve sore throats and enhance immunity. Used by some herbalists to relieve some menopausal symptoms due to oestrogenic properties. Sage may also reduce milk flow during lactation—so avoid during breastfeeding. Do not use if you are pregnant.

Thyme herb - Useful for ear, nose, throat, and chest infections. (may be combined with other herbs). One of the strongest herbal antiseptics. Useful to combat coughs and colds in children. Avoid in pregnancy.

Here is a useful way of using thyme for coughs and colds from www.nimh.org.uk

"Are you starting with the symptoms of a cold? At the first sign of a sore throat, cough, or stuffy nose many herbalists recommend sipping a hot tea made from fresh thyme to help you to feel better quickly.

Scrunch up a few sprigs of fresh thyme from the garden or your local supermarket and put them in a small teapot. Add freshly boiled water and put the lid on to keep in the steam and the volatile oils it contains.

Allow your tea to infuse for at least ten minutes before straining it into a cup and adding a slice of unwaxed lemon with the peel included. You can add a spoonful of honey to sweeten your tea if you like, as this can also help to soothe a sore throat. If you feel a bit shivery, then a small slice of fresh ginger root added to your cup of thyme tea will help to warm you up and dispel any chills you may have.

Gently sip your hot tea, whilst breathing in the aromatic vapours. This soothing traditional remedy can be drunk three times a day as required."
Suggested by Medical Herbalist Phil Deakin

Herbal teas are generally safe to use but should not replace medical treatment. If you are unsure whether a herb is safe for you or wish to know more about Herbal Medicine, ask your local Medical Herbalist. To find a qualified Herbalist near to you, see www.nimh.org.uk

AFTERWORD

The information in this book is a collection of some of the knowledge kindly imparted to me by others. If there are errors, they are due to my own misunderstanding and not that of my teachers. I have chosen the mode of presentation similar to the methods and ideas that have benefited me, my family, my fellow Tai Chi practitioners and my patients over the years. The methods and ideas presented are not definitive or conclusive, there will certainly be others that are more appropriate for you and so you should investigate them further. As a starting point you might wish to access some of the texts listed in the bibliography.

Thank you for purchasing this book, I hope that you enjoy using the information and that you gain some benefit from it.

Very best wishes for your future health and happiness,

Peter.

This book was sponsored by

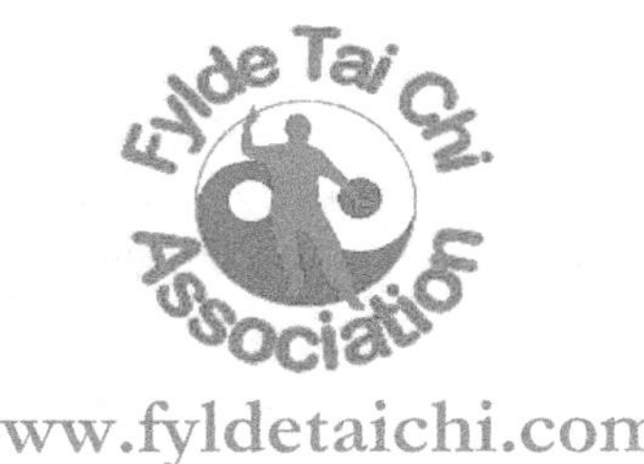

www.fyldetaichi.com

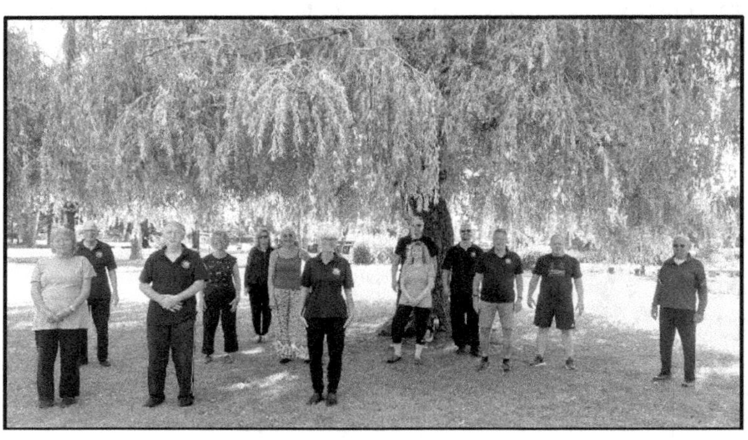

Some members of Fylde Tai Chi Association absorbing the chi of a weeping willow, following "Tai Chi in the Park" on a beautiful, sunny, summer Sunday morning.

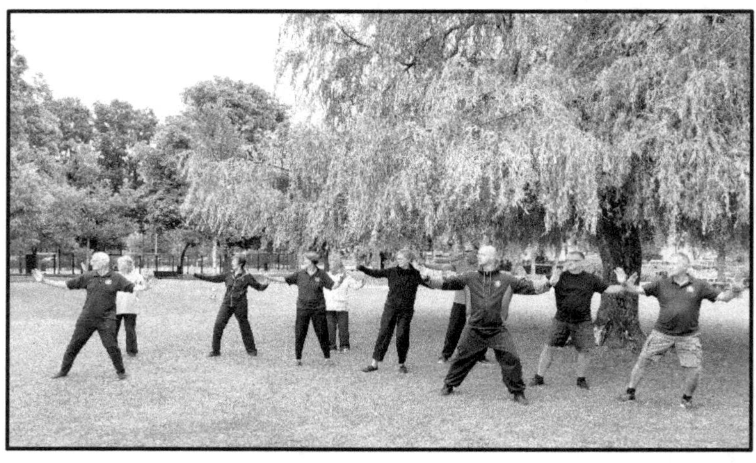

Some members of Fylde Tai Chi Association practising Sun Style Tai Chi on a beautiful, but not so sunny, summer Sunday morning in Poulton le Fylde Park

BIBLIOGRAPHY

BERK, W.R. (1989) Chinese Healing Arts, Internal Kung Fu. USA: Unique Publications.

CARTMELL, T. (2003) A Study of Taijiquan by Sun Lutang. USA: North Atlantic Books

CHENG MANCHING and SMITH, R.W. (1967) Tai-Chi. Vermont: Tuttle

DA LIU (1974) Tai Chi Chuan and I Ching. London: Routledge and Kegan Paul Ltd

DOCHERTY, D. (1997) Complete Tai Chi Chuan. UK: The Crowood Press Ltd

DOCHERTY, D. (2015) The Complete Tai Chi Tutor. UK: Gaia Publications.

FARRELL, J&P. (2017) Understanding Chi Kung. 2nd edition. USA: CreateSpace Independent Publishing

FRANTZIS, B.K. (1993) Opening the Energy Gates of Your Body. USA: North Atlantic Books

FRANTZIS, B.K. (2006) Tai Chi: Health for Life. USA: North Atlantic Books

HOBDAY, R. (1999) The Healing Sun. UK: Findhorn Publications

KAM CHUEN. L. (1991) The Way of Energy. New York: Simon and Schuster

KAPTCHUK, T.D. (1983) Chinese Medicine: The Web That Has No Weaver. p35-41. UK: Rider Publications.

LAMA JAMPA THAYE (2018) (https://soundcloud.com/lama-jampa-thaye/the-power-of-buddhism-bodhichitta-and-the-six-perfections)

LIANG, S.Y and WU, C.W (1993) A Guide to Taijiquan. USA: YMAA Publications

LO, B *et al* **(1979)** The Essence of Tai Chi Chuan. USA: North Atlantic Books

MAOSHING, N. (1995) The Yellow Emperor's Classic of Internal Medicine. USA: Shambala.

OLSEN, S.A. (1992) The Jade Emperor's Mind Seal Classic. USA: Dragon Door Publications.

PETERSON, J.B. (2018) 12 Rules for Life. UK: Penguin.

SWAIN, L. (2005) The Essence and Applications of Taijiquan by Yang Chengfu. USA: North Atlantic Books

TORTURA, G.J. and GRABOWSKI, S.R. (1996) Principles of Anatomy and Physiology, 8th Edition. USA: Harper and Collins.

WILLIAMS, T. (1995) Chinese Medicine. Dorset: Element Books.

YANG, J. M. (1988) Eight Pieces of Brocade. USA: YMAA Publications.

YANG, J. M. (1989) Muscle / Tendon Changing and Marrow Brain-Washing Chi Kung. USA: YMAA Publications.

YANG, J. M. (1990) The Essence of Tai Chi Kung. USA: YMAA Publications.

YANG, J. M. (1990) Muscle / Tendon Changing and Marrow Brain-Washing Chi Kung. USA: YMAA Publications.

YANG, J. M. (2014) Tai Chi Qigong: The Internal Foundation of Tai Chi Chuan. USA: YMAA Publications.

YUDKIN, J. (2016) Pure, White and Deadly: How Sugar Is Killing Us and What We Can Do to Stop It. UK: Penguin

ABOUT THE AUTHOR

Peter has studied and practised Gung fu, including Tai Chi and Chi Gung for almost half a century. Since first learning Peking Tai Chi, a standardised form of Yang Tai Chi, from Miss Rose Li in the early 70s he has studied other forms with various teachers: most notably Sun Style internal arts from Master Bob Melia, his teachers, Master Lei Shi Tai and Sifu Dave Martin, a first-generation student of the late Grandmaster Sun Jian Yun. In addition to Tai Chi, he has studied Wing Chun Gung Fu and Chu Gar Hung Kuen and Chi Gung under the guidance of his brother, Master John Farrell, the senior student of Grandmaster Chu Shiu Woon.

He holds honours degrees in Health Science and Herbal Medicine. Prior to retirement, he lectured in Human Physiology and other Biosciences at *Blackpool and the Fylde College*, and in addition, for several years there, gave non-vocational tuition in Tai Chi. He continues to teach Tai Chi and Chi Gung for the *Fylde Tai Chi Association* of which he is a founding member, along with his senior student Martin Brady and other Tai Chi stalwarts.

Peter is a Consulting Medical Herbalist (retired) trained under the auspices of *The National Institute of Medical Herbalists*, of which he remains a member. As a Medical Herbalist, he incorporated bodywork modalities such as Chi Gung, Tai Chi and associated techniques as an important part of his treatments. For several years he lectured in clinical examination skills to trainee Medical Herbalist and Homoeopaths at the *University of Central Lancashire*.

He is author of *Limitations in Current Theories of Understanding Bereavement and Grief* published in *Counselling* and *Counselling Reader*, and *Qigong: A Scientific Perspective*, published in *Qi Journal*. He is co-author of *Understanding Chi Kung* and author of *Tai Chi for You*; *Clinical Examination Routines, Common Signs and Symptoms* and *Support of Health and Wellbeing: Rational Disease Resistance*.

Peter is a strong advocate ("*ad nauseam*" - his words) for personal responsibility for health and a pro-active approach to healthcare. As part of this approach, he is proud to be able to pass on experience and knowledge gained over almost half a century of study and practise, being, in his words, solely the result of the kindness of his wonderful teachers.

Other books by the author

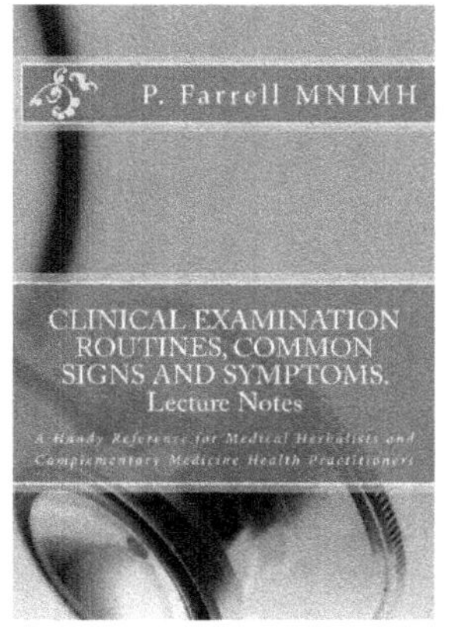

"A convenient reference and general guide to basic orthodox clinical examination routines, along with identification of some common signs and symptoms."

ISBN-13: 978-1543152432

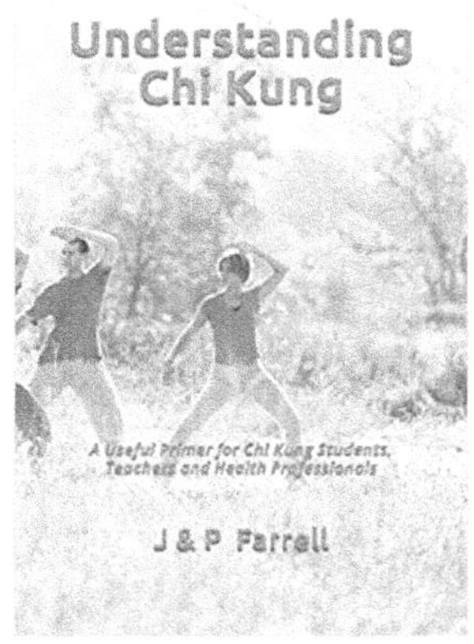

"A useful primer for beginners and experienced Chi Kung practitioners, teachers and health professionals."

ISBN-13: 979-8663125086

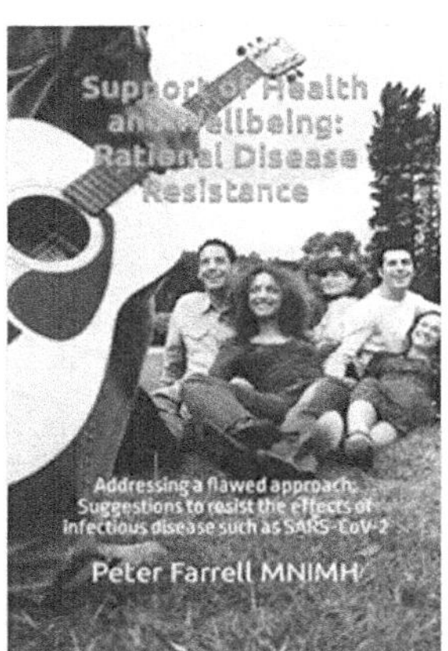

" A must read for those who require a rational understanding and courageous approach to infectious disease resistance.

The author encourages a long-term strategy of a fearless and personally responsible approach to supporting health and well-being to help combat disease assault."

ISBN-13: 979-8474389059